# THE NEW WOMEN'S HEALTH HANDBOOK

## EDITED BY NANCY MACKEITH
illustrated by Kathy Wyatt

*Virago*

London

Published by VIRAGO Limited 1978     Reprinted 1978
4th Floor, 5 Wardour Street
London W1V 3HE

ISBN 0 86068 034 7
Printed in Great Britain by Unwin Brothers, Old Woking, Surrey

VIRAGO is a feminist publishing company:

*'It is only when women start to organize
in large numbers that we become a
political force, and begin to move towards
the possibility of a truly democratic society
in which every human being can be brave,
responsible, thinking and diligent in the struggle
to live at once freely and unselfishly'*

Sheila Rowbotham, *Women, Resistance and Revolution*

**VIRAGO ADVISORY GROUP**

Carol Adams                  Christine Jackson
Sally Alexander              Suzanne Lowry
Anita Bennett                Jean McCrindle
Liz Calder                   Mandy Merck
Bea Campbell                 Cathy Porter
Angela Carter                Spare Rib Collective
Mary Chamberlain             Mary Stott
Deirdre Clark                Anne Summers (Australia)
Anna Coote                   Rosalie Swedlin
Jane Cousins                 Michelene Wandor
Anna Davin                   Alison Weir
Rosalind Delmar              Elizabeth Wilson
Zoe Fairbairns               Women in Education
Carolyn Faulder              Barbara Wynn

# CONTENTS

## PREFACE TO SECOND EDITION

This is the second edition of the Women's Health Handbook, first published in 1976. We have rewritten some chapters and corrected errors but learning about women's health care is a continuous process and we hope you will keep up to date by reading (addresses of women's papers are at the back of the book); or better still, join a health group!

This edition comes out at a time when women are being hit by cuts in the National Health Service. While drug manufacturers are still raking in profits we are losing jobs and being expected to provide the same care at home for free. We hope this book is helpful to women on a practical level and also to those working on many fronts for a healthier service.

ACKNOWLEDGEMENTS

Thanks to Sarah Haynes, Miranda Miller, Stephanie Munro, Agnes Pivot, Lee Sanders, Terry Wragg, Ruth Todasco, Sandra Allen, Christine Beels, Lee Sanders, Jan Wallis, Feminist Books.

# INTRODUCTION

*Nancy, why are we doing this handbook?*

We need a British handbook mainly because previous women's health literature has been about America and there hasn't been much information on how to use a speculum or what you see when you do use one.

*How does self examination help us?*

Self examination helps you to think of your body as basically healthy. When you look round the group most people are well; it is not a case of looking around and seeing what is wrong with everybody; there is probably only one person who is ill in any group. Then if you study yourself say once a week over some time, you can learn your own cycle, learn that extra secretion at one point does not necessarily mean that you have caught something. It may mean that your period is coming soon or that you are ovulating. You learn how wide the normal spectrum is and you learn what is normal for you as well as what is abnormal. It demystifies what doctors are looking at when they put speculums in; for me that was the most exciting thing, just to realize what they were looking at. It is important that in this book we make it quite clear that self examination isn't eccentric. It has a very important political history. The changeover from being a sort of barber's surgeon technician to the present day doctor who makes moral judgments is very recent and very threatening. Dr Peter Diggory who runs an out-patient abortion clinic said once that any GP can do an abortion and any policeman can do an out-patient vacuum abortion. He picks a male paramedic because he knows that the uterus is the battleground where women must fight to regain control. For instance, the chart on page 4 was taken from a US Family Planning journal and shows clearly how women's struggle to control their bodies and their fertility is a political struggle.

*How do self help groups start?*

Usually with someone who has done it before showing women how to use a speculum. Members of the group may all have something in common — perhaps recent childbirth. The Swansea Guide to having a baby grew out of that group's experiences. Another group might do pregnancy testing and referral. Some people can attack what they have been doing already with renewed commitment because they have new knowledge and confidence. They might go back to their abortion campaign because they

1

finally realise how important it is to have an abortion under 12 weeks. Up to now people have been very interested in getting abortion and contraception on demand. Now they seem to be much more interested in the quality of the care they are getting. As well as actually getting the abortion, they want it to be a good one. They want to be able to have kids afterwards and they also want to know what is happening to them much more. Doctors still give out contraceptives that are very unsuitable. So we have to watch out for ourselves because the doctors are not doing it for us.

Contraception is a 'medical' problem; every magazine you read says 'Go to your doctor'. Women go to the doctor and he says 'Here is the pill, dear' and they go away without even having their blood pressure or medical history taken. Only 10 per cent of GPs now practising have any contraception training. This is worrying because the responsibility is now more and more with GPs.

*What else is in the book besides self examination, contraception and abortion?*

We do give a detailed description of the reproductive cycle although we don't go into pregnancy and birth as they need another book! We have included such common problems as infertility and vaginal discharge.

*Can self help groups do diagnosis and treatment?*

You can pick up problems early — you can say when something began in relation to other factors like whether a red patch on your cervix was there before you got your IUD. The only things we treat at the moment are thrush and trichomoniasis. We could do far more if we had culture and microscope facilities; taking pap smears, for example, would be no problem.

*What about the general non-specific things like an itchy vagina?*

Well, a lot of that would be thrush and we could do a lot to help the woman by asking her if she's on the pill or antibiotics, going over her diet, seeing if she eats too much sugar or something else which exacerbates thrush. Careful groups should be able to find that out whereas a busy GP might miss it. Then, as well as telling you how to examine your breasts we talk about cancer and the presently available treatments. We talk about smoking because women are now more likely to get cancer of the lung than of the cervix. So that you get an idea of the structures that govern our health care, we have included sections on Social Security and the National Health Service (NHS). The biggest gap in the book is sexuality.

We do have a terrific heterosexual bias because of the information on reproduction. We only have small sections on nutrition and women and psychiatry. They deserve a book for each of them. We hope nevertheless that this book serves as a starting point to help women fight for better health care.

**Table 1. Examples of Proposed Measures to Reduce U.S. Fertility, by Universality or Selective Impact:**

| Universal Impact | Selective Impact Depending on Socio-Economic Status | | Measures Predicated on Existing Motivation to Prevent Unwanted Pregnancy |
|---|---|---|---|
| Social Contraints | Economic Deterrents/Incentives | Social Controls | |
| Restructure family: <br> a) Postpone or avoid marriage <br> b) Alter image of ideal family size | Modify tax policies: <br> a) Substantial marriage tax <br> b) Child tax <br> c) Tax married more than single <br> d) Remove parents' tax exemption <br> e) Additional taxes on parents with more than 1 or 2 children in school | Compulsory abortion of out-of-wedlock pregnancies <br><br> Compulsory sterilization of all who have two children except for a few who would be allowed three | Payments to encourage con-traception <br><br> Payments to encourage abortion |
| Compulsory education of children | | | Allow certain contraceptives to be distributed non-medically |
| Encourage increased homo-sexuality | Reduce/eliminate paid maternity leave or benefits | Confine childbearing to only a limited number of adults | |
| Educate for family limitation | Reduce/eliminate children's or family allowances | Stock certificate-type permits for children | Improve contraceptive technology |
| Fertility control agents in water supply | Bonuses for delayed marriage and greater child-spacing | | Make contraception truly available and accessible to all |
| Encourage women to work | Pensions for women of 45 with less than N children | Housing Policies: <br> a) Discouragement of private home ownership <br> b) Stop awarding public housing based on family size | Improve maternal health care, with family planning as a core element |
| | Eliminate Welfare payments after first 2 children | | |
| | Chronic Depression | | |
| | Require women to work and provide few child care facilities | | |
| | Limit/eliminate public-financed medical care, scholarships, housing, loans and subsidies to families with more than N children | | |

Source: Frederick S. Jaffe, "Activities Relevant to the Study of Population Policy for the U.S.," Memorandum to Bernard Berelson, March 11, 1969.

# BASIC SELF EXAMINATION

The intention of self examination is to familiarize a woman with those parts of her body with which she has been denied familiarity. Underlying this is a responsibility for keeping her body healthy, a responsibility which a woman can choose to undertake herself, rather than abdicate to a doctor. This involves becoming conscious of the well body, so that she becomes sensitive to changes in her body which might indicate the development of sickness.

When this is applied to most parts of the body, this theory is more or less taken for granted. We see our faces every morning in the mirror and touch them many times during the day. So we soon become aware of a swelling developing into a spot, or a change in colour or temperature. And yet when this is applied to the genitals many people react negatively. They see it as a sexual perversion and an obscene interest in 'private parts'. To some people a woman knowing her cervix and her vagina is too powerful a tool for her to cope with. Using a speculum, she might get an infection or damage herself, or she might get dangerously frightened or worried by what she sees. Or it might threaten her relationship with the medical profession. She might diagnose herself and not go to the doctor and the infection may get worse; she might waste the doctor's time by wanting to discuss and question what she has seen. And anyway, what's the point when she can go to the doctor and he'll look for her and tell her if there's anything she needs to know.

Our answer to these attitudes is that a doctor does not see you often enough to know what is normal for you. He cannot be sensitive to the subtle changes that would enable him to practise preventive medicine by detecting early signs of infections, disease and pregnancy. With a few exceptions the medical profession is often evasive and condescending and doctors do not tell us what we want to know.

The politics of self help are a challenge to the medical profession's attitude to our bodies; and they are also a challenge to the taboos which surround our reproductive organs, which alienate us from our genitals as being unmentionable, and under most circumstances, untouchable. Whereas in fact the genitals are an important functioning part of the body which we need to keep healthy. It is on that level that we learn to relate to ourselves through self examination.

To undertake self examination is a conscious decision because you need to use a certain amount of equipment; you need a light source, a mirror, a speculum, and water or a water-soluble vaginal jelly such as KY jelly. (Don't use vaseline, it's not water soluble and it affects the natural balance in the vagina.) Keep your speculum clean by washing it with warm water and soap, and store it in a clean place. Practise opening and closing the speculum before using it, clicking the ratchet into position to hold the blades open.

Empty your bladder and find a position which is comfortable for you and where you are warm and undisturbed. Start by looking at the outer organs with a mirror. The first thing you will see is the outer genitals or *vulva.* The pubic hair grows from the outer lips (*labia majora*) and the pubis. As you look more closely you will see the *clitoris,* a smooth pink bump (you may need to pull back the folds of skin which cover it). This is richly supplied with nerves and plays an important part in orgasm. If you are not sure where it is, feel for it, it is the most sensitive part of your genitals. The hood which covers the shaft of the clitoris is part of the inner lips (*labia minora*) which extend from the clitoris to frame the sides of the vaginal opening. Then spread the lips and look at the vaginal and urinary openings. The urinary opening is much smaller than the vaginal opening just between the clitoris and the vagina. Feel for swellings in the *Bartholins glands* (two small rounded bodies on either side of the vaginal opening). They can occasionally become infected, but you will not ordinarily feel them unless they are swollen. Once you become familiar with these parts you can look for changes in colour, irritations, bumps and swellings.

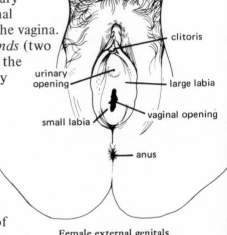

Female external genitals

Then move on to examine your interior genitals. Use a speculum to spread the vaginal walls to get a view of the *cervix.* Find the most comfortable position for you to insert the speculum, maybe think of it like putting in a tampon. Some women lie with their knees bent up, some squat, some stand with one leg on the table or bed. Judge it according to your own comfort and use lubrication if you like. Breath deeply, relax and don't rush yourself. Always insert the speculum closed so that you don't pinch the skin on the walls of the vagina. Insert it so that the handle is pointing off to the side, and slide it in as far as it will go. Then turn it so that the handle is pointing up, open the speculum, (as you will have practised) and fasten it. You can also put the speculum in with the handles facing upwards. Hold the mirror in front of the vagina and shine the light into it so that it reflects into the vagina and you can see inside.

The *vagina,* (birth canal) extends inwards from the bladder

6

and the rectum at a 45° angle to the floor when you are standing. The walls of the vagina are pink in colour and textured. The volume of the vagina is potential, not actual; women are not a series of holes. The elasticity of the vaginal skin is due to the folds, which flatten out as the vagina expands in intercourse or childbirth. The colour and texture will vary among women and during the menstrual cycle.

At the end of the vagina you can see the cervix, a smooth, shiny, pink, dome-shaped protrusion. The cervix is the narrow part of the *uterus* (womb), a thick-walled, muscular organ in the lower abdomen between the bladder and the rectum. A non-pregnant uterus is about the size of a walnut. The uterus changes position during the menstrual cycle and so the cervix can shift position. If you can't see the cervix, try inserting the speculum at a different angle, and pull in your stomach and massage downwards. Breath deeply and relax — don't worry, it's there somewhere. The size and colour of the cervix will vary, affected by pregnancy, age, and the time of the menstrual cycle.

In the centre of the cervix is the *os*, or opening to the uterus. This also will vary in size and shape. It is usually round in women who have had no children and slit-shaped and larger in those who have. If you have an IUD (see chapter on Intra-uterine Devices) you will see the string coming from the os. Note the secretions within the vagina. Secretions and mucus are normal, vary with each woman, and change during the menstrual cycle. With increased oestrogen before ovulation there is a sharp drop in the calcium content of the mucus and many women have noted that the mucus becomes clear and stringy. After ovulation, under the influence of progesterone, the mucus becomes thicker and dryer.

plastic speculum — handles up

cervix

os

anus

Take your time examining yourself, and when you have finished, remove the speculum leaving the blades open; to close them would pinch the walls of the vagina. Pull the speculum out of the vagina, and smell the mucus on the speculum, as this will be useful in determining infections. The speculum should be washed and kept clean.

If you keep a journal of what you can see during self examination, you will have a record to refer to, and over the months you will be able to check which changes are normal and recurring and which are unusual. Making drawings can be helpful to record sizes, shapes, and positions.

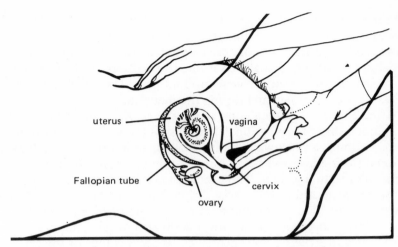

uterus

vagina

Fallopian tube

cervix

ovary

Women in health groups can also learn how to do internal exams —
feeling the size and position of the uterus. Pregnancy can be felt at
about 8 weeks from the date of the last period — the uterus will be
softer and larger. This uterus is about 12 weeks pregnant.

Here are some suggestions of things to look for from the San Francisco
Women's Health Centre:

*Vulva:* colour of outer lips; colour of inner lips; clitoris: Bartholins glands
—not normally seen or felt unless infected.

*Vaginal Walls:* hymen — sometimes seen about an inch in; colour of walls;
texture — firm, puffy, ridged, smooth; surface: clean, tender, any
discharge.

*Discharge:* colour — clear, milky white, yellow, greenish. smell: yeasty,
fishy, acidic, bland. consistency: thick, thin, stringy, foamy, chunky.
amount: profuse, moderate, small.

*Cervix:* colour: pink, red, blueish, discolourations: red patches, bumps;
position of cervix.

*Os:* shape: dimple, slit, size: open, closed, usual shape. (IUD string length).

*Mucous Secretion from Os:* colour, consistency: thick, thin, stringy; smell,
amount.

*Menstrual Blood:* colour, amount.

*General Health Information:* ease of speculum insertion; on or off pill,
IUD in or removed, painful intercourse, day of cycle.

| Date of | Vulva | Vaginal Walls | Cervix | Os | Secretion from Os | Discharge | Point in Cycle | General Health |
|---|---|---|---|---|---|---|---|---|
| 1st weekly examination | | | | | | | | |
| 2nd week | | | | | | | | |
| 3rd week | | | | | | | | |
| 4th week | | | | | | | | |
| 5th week | | | | | | | | |
| 6th week | | | | | | | | |

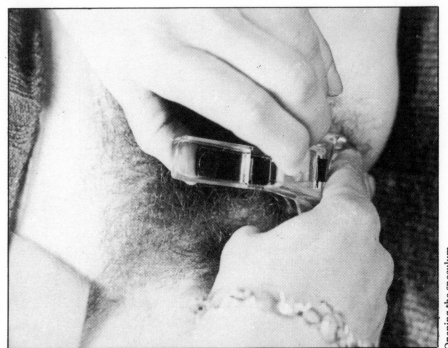

Opening the speculum

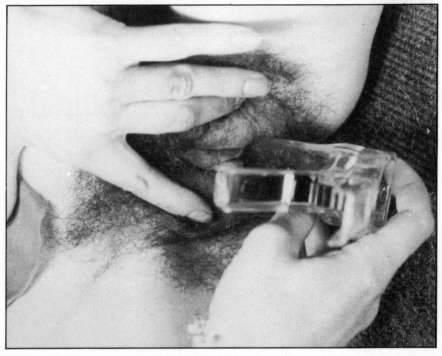

Inserting the speculum

10

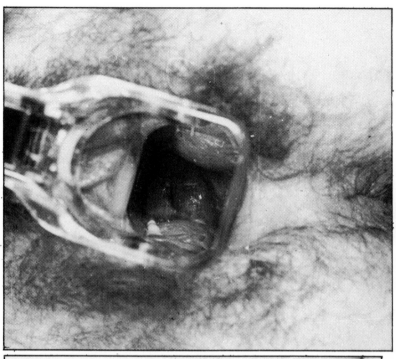

This woman has never been pregnant so her os is quite small. Her cervix in this photo is tilted upwards so the back of her uterus will be towards her spine. This position is called 'retroverted' and a retroverted uterus is sometimes blamed for painful periods, sterility etc, but the healthy uterus moves around all the time and anyway sperm can swim round corners. Her cervix is very healthy, firm, pink and shiny.

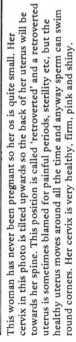

This woman has had one abortion so her os has been dilated a little. You can see how it would be slightly easier to put an IUD in her but it is important to dilate as little as possible when putting instruments into the uterus (see chapters on Abortion and IUDs) so as not to damage the narrow cervical canal.

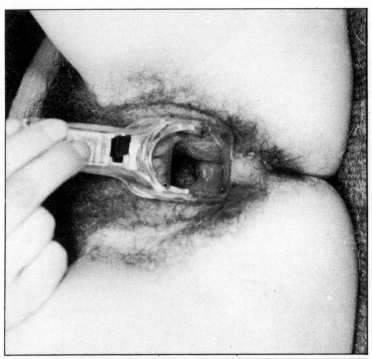

This woman has had a child. She has a red patch above the os. The cells which grow inside the cervical canal are redder than the outside ones. Sometimes these red cells grow outside and this is called an erosion. (see Cancer chapter for explanation of erosions and pap smears.) Like all the women in these photos she is healthy and with her speculum she can keep an eye on the erosion and seek treatment when necessary, for example if she noticed a discharge.

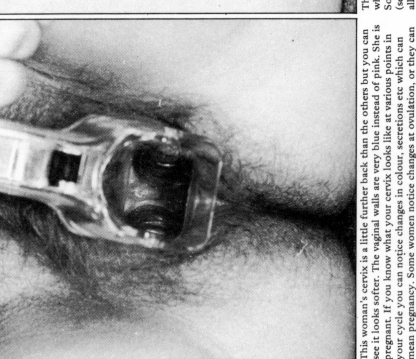

This woman's cervix is a little further back than the others but you can see it looks softer. The vaginal walls are very blue instead of pink. She is pregnant. If you know what your cervix looks like at various points in your cycle you can notice changes in colour, secretions etc which can mean pregnancy. Some women notice changes at ovulation, or they can spot an infection before it gets to be a nuisance. In each woman these signs will be different, so know yourself.

# BREAST SELF EXAMINATION

When you examine your breasts, you are looking for changes that may have occurred in them since the last time you looked. Therefore you need to look regularly, so you get used to the feel of yourself, and it's also best to use the same time each month — just after a period and ideally on the same day of each cycle. The changes could be in the shape or size of the breast or nipple, changes in skin texture, puckering of the nipple or skin around it, discharge from the nipple, swelling of the upper arm or armpit. These changes you can best observe by looking in a mirror with your arms raised over your head. When you do the rest of the examination, which will involve feeling for thickening or lumps, it's best to lie down, in a warm atmosphere if possible, with a small pillow, or cushion to put under the shoulder of the breast you're feeling. This helps the breast tissue to spread out. Use your right hand for your left breast and raise the left arm above your head. Use the flat fleshy part of your hand (keeping your fingers together) or use your fingertips. Press gently on, first, the lower outer quarter of your breast. Next the lower inner quarter, then the upper inner quarter and lastly the upper outer quarter. As you lower your arm feel under the armpit. Then repeat on the other side.

A lump may be quite soft, or definitely hard, or slightly moving beneath your fingers. It may also be a soft, massy thickening of the whole area. A normal breast feels quite soft and squashy when pressed, as breasts are made up only of fatty tissue and only have a little muscle at the top. If you do see or feel anything different to last month's examination, or anything that you are doubtful about, it's best to go straight to the doctor. Almost always these changes are not indicative of anything serious, but if there is a malignancy your speed in detecting it and taking prompt action could be of great importance.

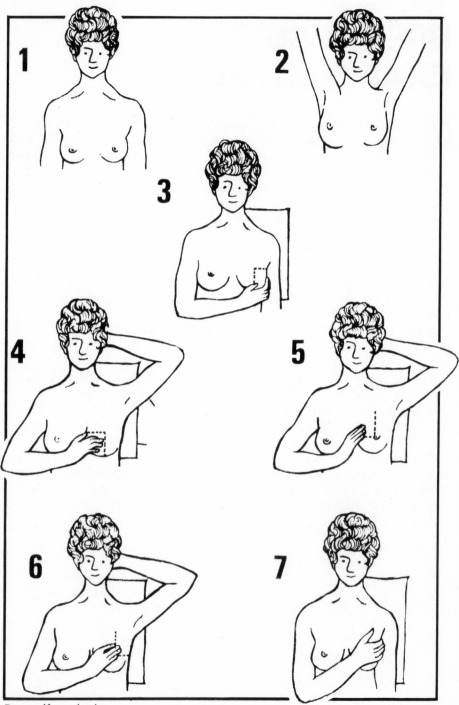

Breast self examination

# THE MENSTRUAL CYCLE

At some point between the ages of 10 and 18 (the common age in this country is about 13), we start to have 'periods'. We probably know beforehand that having periods means that we will bleed for a few days roughly every month, and that the process is something to do with eggs and babies! We might also be frightened of having pain with our periods because of having observed mothers, elder sisters, girls at school etc. We might wonder why periods are sometimes called 'having the curse'. We might actually have a lot of pain, go to the GP, and be told that the pain is quite normal and that it will go away when we have babies (the assumption being that at some point in time we will have babies). What few of us have explained to us is the mechanism of menstruation — what processes are actually going on in our bodies. Most of us remain in the somewhat mystified state of having confused ideas linking periods, pain and babies not only to the fact of being 'biologically female', but also the state of being 'sociologically female'.[1]    As soon as we realize that this confusion exists we can *start* untangling it by understanding how our biological selves work. What follows here is a brief account, firstly of the particular parts of our bodies concerned with the menstrual cycle, and secondly, how the menstrual cycle is controlled by hormones. For fuller accounts see the references below.

The parts of our bodies concerned with the menstrual cycle are:

1) The *hypothalamus*

2) The *pituitary*

3) The *ovaries*

4) The *endometrium*

The *hypothalamus* is a special part of the brain, which working with the pituitary, controls the stages of the menstrual cycle.

The *pituitary* is a very small gland, situated at the base of the brain (immediately below the hypothalamus) and has been called the 'master' gland of the body, since the hormones it manufactures affect almost all the other glands and organs in the body. As noted above, the pituitary is itself controlled by the hypothalamus. The hypothalamus produces substances (not known why) which are called *releasing factors* which then stimulate the pituitary gland to release hormones into the general circulation. The hormones concerned with the menstrual cycle are known as the *gonadotrophins* (those which affect the ovaries *gonads*) and there are two of them, these being:

1) *follicle stimulating hormone* (FSH)

2) *luteinising hormone* (LH)

The *ovaries* at birth contain the *follicles* (cells) which are to become the egg-cells *(ova)*. Only a certain number of follicles are present in each ovary — numbers from various sources range from 40,000 - 400,000. The ovaries also produce two hormones concerned with the menstrual cycle. They are known as the female sex hormones and are:

1) *Oestrogen*

2) *Progesterone*

The *endometrium* is the lining membrane of the uterus. It is composed of narrow tubes *(endometrial glands)* set in several layers of cells *(endometrial stromal cells)*. It is acted upon by the oestrogen and progesterone from the ovary which prepare it to nourish a fertilized egg. If no fertilized egg implants itself into the lining, then it is shed, and the shedding of the unwanted endometrium is called menstruating or having a period.

These then are the particular parts of our bodies concerned with the menstrual cycle; to understand the processes of ovulation and menstruation, we must understand how the whole cycle is controlled by hormones. The menstrual cycle is an ongoing and complicated process. A complete cycle includes the days when bleeding occurs plus the days before bleeding occurs again — cycles varying in length from 20-36 days with 28 days being considered the average. It is for convenience that we consider the day we start bleeding as the first day of a cycle and therefore the day *before* we start bleeding as the *last* day of a cycle.

On the first day of the cycle, when we are bleeding, our bodies are preparing for the following month. The hypothalamus is sending quantities of the FSH-releasing factor to stimulate the cells in the pituitary which secrete (manufacture) FSH. The level of FSH rises in the blood and stimulates about 12-20 of the egg follicles in the ovary. It is not known at this time why only certain follicles respond to the influence of FSH or why (usually) only one follicle is stimulated to ovulation [2]. As the follicles grow, they manufacture oestrogen, and by 13 days after the cycle began the level of oestrogen in the blood has increased six times above the level at the beginning. The rising blood level of oestrogen has a 'feed-back' effect on the hypothalamus — that is the oestrogen level rises, so the FSH releasing factor is reduced, the hypothalamus sending instead quantities of the other substance called the LH-releasing factor to

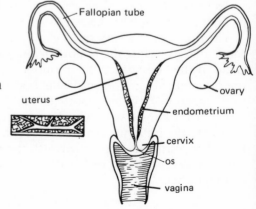

stimulate the cells in the pituitary which secrete (manufacture) LH. Under the influence of the FSH, one follicle has by now grown the most and has moved through the ovary to reach its surface, where it makes a very small bulge which can be seen with the naked eye. Under the influence of the FSH, the follicle bursts (ovulation) and the egg is pushed out. The released egg is caught by the finger-like (fimbrial) ends of the Fallopian tube and begins its 6½-day journey to the uterus, moved along by contractions of the Fallopian tube. If fertilization is to occur, it normally takes place in the outer third of the tube. If not, it disintegrates, and is sloughed off in vaginal secretions, usually before bleeding occurs.

After the egg has been released, the ruptured follicle collapses and the LH acts on the cells of its walls, turning them yellow. The collapsed follicle is now called the *corpus luteum* (yellow body). The cells in the corpus luteum continue to secrete oestrogen. The other stimulated follicles which failed to complete development, gradually degenerate, but before they die, they too secrete small amounts of oestrogen. The cells in the corpus luteum also manufacture a new hormone, *progesterone.* If the egg is not fertilized, the corpus luteum degenerates about 12 days after the follicle ruptured, because of another feed-back mechanism. The rising pro-gesterone level inhibits the pituitary secretion of LH. As the corpus luteum degenerates with the reduction of LH, the levels of oestrogen and proges-terone in the blood fall, having two effects: the restraint on the FSH is stimulating the follicles and the growing follicles are manufactur-ing oestrogen, as well as causing a decline in FSH and a rise in LH, the oestrogen stimulates the endo-metrium, which, as we have seen, is the lining membrane of the ut-erus. Oestrogen makes the endo-metrial glands grow longer, the stromal cells become larger, and many blood vessels appear. The endometrium thus increases in thickness and this part of the cycle is called the *proliferative phase.* The addition of proges-terone (produced by the corpus luteum) causes an even greater thickening of the endometrium and induces endometrial glands to secrete a nutritious substance so that a fertilized egg may be

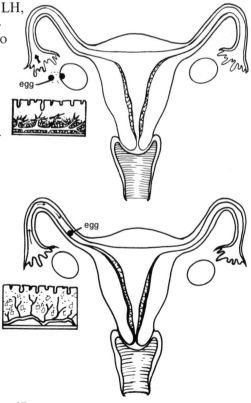

nourished during the time it needs to implant itself into the lining. This part of the cycle is called the *secretory phase* and the stroma become more loosely packed and the blood vessels grow longer. (See Endometrial Biopsy in the Infertility chapter).

However, if the egg has not been fertilized, the oestrogen and progesterone levels in the blood fall, as we have seen, and without the stimulation from these hormones, the endometrium cannot be maintained, and begins to shrink, causing the blood vessels supplying the upper layers of the lining to kink and break. As the cells of these upper layers begin to die from lack of blood, more shrinkage and bleeding occurs and eventually the whole surface is stripped off and shed. This is when bleeding (menstruation) occurs. Lastly, oestrogen and progesterone also affect the cervical mucus. Under the influence of oestrogen, it becomes thinner and wetter, with progesterone it becomes thicker and dryer. The thinness and wetness of the mucus at ovulation (before the progesterone produced by the corpus luteum has affected it) aid the sperms' entrance into the uterus at that time.

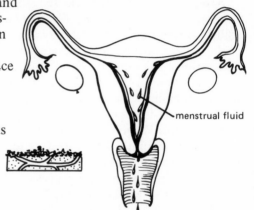

menstrual fluid

## REFERENCES

1 *Sex, Gender and Society*, Ann Oakley, (Temple Smith 1972)
2 *Fundamentals of Obstetrics and Gynaecology*, D. Llewellyn-Jones, (Faber & Faber 1972)

# PERIOD PAINS

From some of the available literature one would think that all women
from the dawn of time have had 28-day menstrual cycles, but this has not
always been the case. If you conceived soon after beginning menstruation
and breastfed each child for several years you would only have a few
periods. This partly explains why some cultures have taboos about menstruation – it is an unusual event. Very irregular periods are a problem if you
are trying to get pregnant because you are not ovulating as often as other
women, but heavy periods can make you anaemic (the blood lacks iron
and you feel tired all the time). Some women also experience tension and/
or pain. According to Katherina Dalton, who wrote *The Menstrual Cycle*,
there are 2 main types of period pain (known as *dysmenorrhoea*) –
congestive and spasmodic.

## CONGESTIVE

The symptoms are pre-menstrual tension (bloated feeling; irritability;
tiredness; clumsiness; greasy hair; spots): on arrival of the period, low
backache and some pain – nagging rather than awful. The pains last one or
two days, and many women say that the depression up to the onset of the
period is the worst thing.

The *adrenal glands* (attached to kidneys) produce many *corticosteroids,*
each with a different function. Some are responsible for the water balance
in the tissues of the body, others regulate the sodium and potassium in the
cells, some prevent allergic reactions, others regulate the level of the blood
sugar and some mobilize mechanisms responsible for the protection of the
body from bacterial and viral infections.

In the adrenals progesterone is formed from simpler chemical com-
pounds. The progesterone is the base, from which, after more chemical
reactions the many vital corticosteroids are formed. Thus progesterone is
present in the adrenals throughout the entire monthly cycle and it is the
essential basis for all corticosteroids. The ovary also produces progesterone,
but only during the second half of the monthly cycle, and its production
stops at menstruation.

If, during the second half of the menstrual cycle, the ovary produces
insufficient progesterone for the requirements of the uterus, some progesterone might be taken from the other source, the adrenal glands,
leaving them short for their production of corticosteroids. The balance of
corticosteroids is temporarily upset and may result in water retention
(bloated feeling), imbalance of sodium and potassium, failure to control
allergic reactions, alteration of the blood sugar level and lowered resistance
to infection. All these reactions could account for the presence of the

various symptoms.

Progesterone is insoluble in water and can only be given by injection, so one form of treatment is injections of progesterone every couple of days during the second half of the menstrual cycle. Progestogens are synthetically-produced forms of progesterone. They are water soluble and can be taken by mouth. Birth control pills contain different amounts of progestogens and are used with varying success in the treatment of congestive dysmenorrhoea. Progesterone, oestrogen and androgens (the male sex hormone) have very similar chemical structures. So progestogen taken in contraceptive pills may be used by some women's bodies not only to build the lining of the uterus, but also as an oestrogen or some other hormone – in which case it will cause nausea, weight gain or some other undesirable response. So it's well worth trying several different brands of pill to see if one is effective in bringing relief – although for some women none may be. A few gynaecologists are using *mono oxidase inhibitors* (drugs used in some sorts of depression). We think you shouldn't take these unless you are desperate as they are very strong and you can't eat cheese or drink wine while you are taking them, but some women have found them helpful for severe pre-menstrual depression.

Don't drink too much fluid before your periods and, most important, know your cycle and don't plan to do anything stressful at the time you are least fit for it.

## SPASMODIC

This type of pain is most common between the ages of 15 and 25. It is not usually associated with pre-menstrual tension. The symptoms are that the onset of pain is on the first day of the period although it may continue for the next 2 or 3 days and the pain is most severe on the first day, usually felt as spasms of acute colicky pains in the lower abdomen. These women have an excess of progesterone produced in comparison with oestrogen.

Taking high oestrogen birth control pills for a short time can sometimes help but this has drawbacks (see Pill chapter). Plenty of bed rest, hot water bottles, warm drinks, warm baths can also help. Menstrual extraction may relieve this type of pain. Orgasm relieves the cramps in many women.

Period pains are now also thought to be due to chemicals produced in the blood called *prostaglandins*. These act on the uterus causing spasm and there are tablets to prevent this. Indomethacin (Indoad) is one and Mefanimic acid (marketed as Postan) is another. They are not a good idea if you have gastric ulcers as they may cause bleeding. You take them just as you feel the pain beginning and then 1 or 2 every 4 hours until the danger time is past.

Pain and bleeding can also be a symptom of disease so you should seek investigation if you are not happy. As we are concerned with well women in this book we refer you to gynaecology textbooks (see end of chapter) for detail, but the commonest disorders include:

### Fibroids

Someone may remark during a routine pelvic examination that you probably have a fibroid because your uterus feels 'bulky'. These are non-malignant growths that often produce no symptoms and therefore need no treatment. If they cause heavy bleeding they can be removed by dilatation and curettage.

### Infection

If the lining of the uterus becomes infected (*endometritis*) or there is infection in the Fallopian tubes (*salpingitis*) this can cause pain (see chapter on Venereal Disease).

### Hormonal Upset

Your cycle can be upset, by childbirth or abortion for example, causing bleeding for many days. This problem often responds to hormone therapy. Some seem to improve after a dilatation and curettage (*d&c*) but this has to be balanced out against the risk of damaging the cervix, leading to problems in keeping a pregnancy later on (*cervical incompetence*).

### General Remedies

Exercises   – see *Periods without Pain*, Erna Wright, (Tandem 1971)

Diet       – include iron rich foods such as liver, eggs, greens, yeast and wheat germ.

Yoga
Acupuncture

## FURTHER READING

*The Menstrual Cycle*, Katherina Dalton, (Penguin 1970)

*Obstetric and Gynaecological Nursing*,
Rosemary E. Bailey, (Bailliere Tindall 1975)

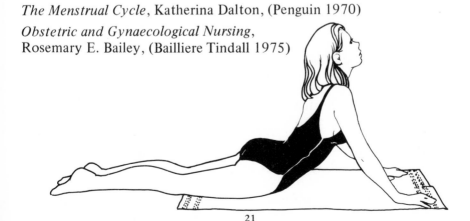

# MENSTRUAL EXTRACTION

A discussion with a woman from a menstrual extraction group.

*What is the history of menstrual extraction and what is it?*
Well, it was developed by Lorraine Rothman of the Feminist Women's Health Centre in Los Angeles. She developed this little device called the Del-um.

*How long ago?*
Four years or so.

*Yes, but what is the Del-um?*
It's a woman controlled way of having a period. It's a safe and simple way of emptying the uterus.

*When do you empty it?*
When you want a period.

*Can you choose your time of the month?*
No, but you can choose to have your period over with in a very short time as opposed to a few days.

*You have to let the lining (of the uterus) build up don't you?*
Yes, and then when the period is due ...

*... you can accelerate it?*
Have it over in a short rather than a long time.

*Wow, do you mean, sorry to keep repeating it, that when you know your period is due, say on a Saturday, you have it on that Saturday and not all the rest of the week as well?*
Yes.

*That's amazing.*
Not even a whole day, it can be 20 minutes.

*Does someone else have to do it? You can't extract yourself?*
Well no, it must be done in a loving, sisterly group.

*That's a bit of a snag isn't it, not to be be able to do it for yourself?*
Well, it's better in a group. It's safer in a group, watching for sterile techniques.

*Because of going into the uterus?*
Yes.

*And done in a group because of all our heavy cultural taboos and things surrounding menstruation?*
Partly, and also because sisterhood is safety and safety is sisterhood.

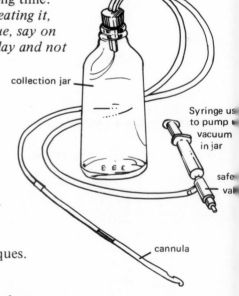

collection jar

Syringe us
to pump
vacuum
in jar

safe

val

cannula

The Del-um —menstrual
extraction kit

*I'd find it very embarrassing to have a period in public. Are other women embarrassed?*
We are socialized to be embarrassed about our periods. If you look through a speculum, the excitement of controlling your period overcomes it. When you know what your period is, that it's cleansing not dirty, that helps. Menstrual extraction in a group breaks down isolation and increases our control.
*Does lots of blood come away?*
Not very much. There has been little research into how much blood women lose with each period, and menstrual extraction groups are taking the trouble to find this out.
*Is there a lot or not as much as you'd think?*
There is variation. Between an eggcupful and half a teacup.
*I find that really helpful — even if I never have it extracted it's going to be good now to have some idea of the quantity. I always feel as though I'm giving away a pint at least every month. Do doctors know about menstrual extraction? Is it used medically?*
There is a little machine, making a vacuum by electrical force, that can take a sample of the monthly lining, to make sure that a woman has no uterine cancer. A few doctors use it but most prefer to give you a general anaesthetic, open the cervix with a dilator and poke around with a curette. It could also be used, this technique, for fertility testing, but they still prefer to gallop in with a curette.
*Do they know that menstrual extraction exists?*
Yes, but they only call it an abortion method. We are not interested in whether sperm is present, we are only interested in controlling our periods. Being mostly male, the doctors only think of sperm in the uterus. They're not interested in women's periods, but only in our bodies as they relate to males, not in our problems.
*You haven't actually said what the Del-um is, what it consists of yet.*
The Del-um kit which consists basically of a collecting jar and tubing, provides a very gentle vacuum source, far more gentle than the electric one used in abortions. Built into the system is a valve which eliminates the risk of an air embolism (bubble of air) entering the uterus.
*Is it safe — really safe?*
In a sisterly set up it's always safe. If you had a problem you could cope with it. I'd be rather worried about it getting into the hands of doctors.
*It sounds as though it's not as safe as having a period, though.*
There is a minute risk of infection, but you only do it on women who are healthy. So far, I've never had any infection trouble.
*Is it natural? Shouldn't we just have our periods?*
This is the first time in history that women have bled so often and so much, because of always being pregnant or breastfeeding and so on before now. The Pill makes us believe we have to bleed once every single month — and doctors have made us think this too.

23

*Does the uterus know it's being emptied differently?*
No, the lining is already in the process of falling off the walls of the uterus. We just remove it in one go.
*Is it legal?*
Under the 1861 Offences Against the Person Act it is 'illegal' to perform an abortion whether or not the woman is pregnant but there hasn't yet been a prosecution involving menstrual extraction.
*Are lots of women already using this method, and just quietly getting on with it?*
It's widely used in America, and here in Britain and the rest of Europe the movement is growing steadily.

# THE MENOPAUSE

At the Sheffield Women & Health Converence (1974), Angela Roddaway from Bristol who joined the women's movement when she was over 50 described how it took her over 6 years to get any discussion group in the movement on the menopause. Women in the movement are always assumed to be fertile - could this be a sub-conscious reflection of the sexist attitude which views older women as cast-offs?

## DEFINITIONS

Literally, the cessation of the monthly process. Ceasing of periods rarely occurs abruptly so generally the whole of the time during which menstruation becomes disrupted is termed the menopause or climacteric. Derogatory definitions include the 'change of life' implying irreversible change in lifestyle.

## WHEN DOES IT OCCUR?

Generally between 35 and 65, average age in Britain 50-51 yrs. Occasionally hysterectomy with removal of the ovaries leads to premature menopause.

## SIZE OF THE PROBLEM

Estimated that 10 million women in Britain are over the age of 45 at any one time.

## IS IT NATURAL?

We are the only known species to live to any significant extent beyond our reproductive years. This is clearly only possible because of our extended life span nowadays.

## WHAT HAPPENS DURING MENOPAUSE?

During the regular menstrual cycle various hormonal changes take place (see chapter on Menstrual Cycle). The menopause begins when the ovaries respond less to pituitary hormones. Less oestrogen and progesterone are produced and fewer and fewer eggs are released until eventually no more are released at all. It is not the case that all the eggs in the ovaries get 'used up'. There are still about 20,000 eggs left at the time of the onset of the menopause. It is simply that the ovaries no longer respond to the messages from the pituitary. It is the drop in the level of oestrogen which is generally responsible for menopausal symptoms.

## MENSTRUATION

Menstrual changes generally follow one of the following patterns:
1) Gradual lessening of flow but periods remain fairly regular.
2) Normal flow but intervals between periods become increasingly longer.
3) Very irregular periods.
4) Sudden complete cessation of periods with no previous changes in flow or regularity.

Occasional heavy periods may occur and this is normal but some abnormal bleeding patterns need medical attention:
1) Increasing and prolonged flow.
2) Very heavy bleeding (flooding) with clots.
3) Spotting or brownish discharge between periods.
4) Bleeding after intercourse.
5) Bleeding many months or years after menstruation has stopped.

The above signs may indicate fibroids or a polyp or, very rarely, cancer. (Fibroids and polyps are non-malignant growths and will quite often be left alone unless you want to get pregnant.)

## CONTRACEPTION

The general rule is to continue using contraception for 1 year after the last period if you are over 50 and for 2 years after your last period if you are under 50.

The Pill: The risks of getting blood clots are greater in older women than in younger women, especially if they smoke, are diabetic, obese or have high blood pressure. It is inadvisable to start on the pill at a menopausal age. It is also difficult to tell if natural periods have ceased because withdrawal bleeding continues on tablet-free weeks.

The IUD may be preferable as it will enable a woman to tell whether or not she is still menstruating. The drawbacks are that the IUD itself may cause heavy bleeding during periods or bleeding between periods. It may exacerbate these conditions if they're already present because of the menopause.

Caps and condoms used with foams and jellies are both useful. They have a lower failure rate in older couples where the woman's fertility may be decreasing.

The rhythm method is even more difficult than before because of irregular periods.

# SYMPTOMS

Menopause is not an illness. It is not invariably accompanied by unpleasant symptoms. Around 15 percent of women pass through the menopause without any unpleasant effects, but 10 per cent suffer from very severe symptoms.

## Hot flushes and sweating

These are the most widely discussed symptoms possibly because they are the most distressing and embarrassing. Generally there is a sensation of feeling very hot which comes on suddenly, usually over the head, neck and shoulders but it may be over the whole body. This is followed by profuse sweating. It generally lasts only 2-3 minutes but in some rare cases, it may last for days. It may start before menstruation ceases but it is most frequent following complete cessation of periods and often lasts for 2-3 years. It generally occurs 2-3 times a day and often at night, sometimes severe enough to wake the woman up.

## Palpitations & dizziness

These are worrying because these symptoms are often associated in the woman's mind with heart trouble. Examination by the GP should exclude these possibilities.

## Gastro intestinal disorders

Flatulence, constipation and abdominal distension. Your GP should also check that there is no major underlying organic disorder causing these.

## Putting on weight

This is generally due to continuing with the same intake of food whilst taking less exercise and can be controlled by diet.

## Insomnia, anxiety, nervousness, tiredness, depression:

In many cases these psychological disturbances are more upsetting than the physical changes. The cause is not entirely understood although they may be relieved by oestrogen therapy. Particular psychological problems experienced depend on individual circumstances but the menopause has a clear universal significance for most women; it underlines advancing age and sharply signals the end of reproductive life and as such could be stressful for some women. Unfortunately, coping with these problems medically all too often hinges on whether the woman has a sympathetic GP who is prepared to spend time exploring the difficulties rather than all too quickly reaching for the prescription pad. Nervousness and irritability are particularly directed at the woman's immediate surrounding family and/or work situation.

## Headaches

These are often more common at this time and are possibly related to hot flushes in that they may be due to the changes taking place in the blood vessels when oestrogen is withdrawn, causing 'vascular headaches' (analagous to headaches occurring just before onset of periods or in tablet-free weeks in women on the Pill).

## Sex

Many women, like Chaucer's wife of Bath, continue to lead a happy, well-adjusted sex life after the menopause. Some however consider that the end of their reproductive life also means an end to their sex life. Others experience an increase in their sex drive which if it is not matched by their partner's can cause problems. The increased interest in sex may be due to freedom from the fear of pregnancy. Both situations can lead to guilt feelings. Lack of variety and sexual imagination can lead to boredom and once interest is lost it is difficult to recover. Sexual problems may be exacerbated by physical changes in the vagina following the withdrawal of oestrogen. The vagina may become dryer than before and be itchy. Due to changes in the acidity of the vagina women are particularly prone to thrush infections. Dryness of the vagina can be overcome by the use of a non-greasy lubricant jelly such as KY jelly. Occasionally the vagina may shrink making intercourse painfully difficult or even impossible. This problem can be overcome by the use of a hormone-containing cream applied locally with or without oral (pills) hormone replacement therapy.

## Osteoporosis

This is a progressively degenerative condition in the bones.
In severe cases it may cause arching of the spine. It explains the higher incidence of broken bones among older women than men. The only treatment is hormone replacement therapy but this cannot reverse any existing osteoporosis. However, if started within three years of the menopause, it does help to decrease the annual 1 percent bone loss seen in untreated women and it also reduces pains in the joints. For some GPs this is the only indication for which they will prescribe HRT in the menopause — other symptoms being regarded as 'trivial' or ones that the patient can put up with!

## HORMONE REPLACEMENT THERAPY (HRT)

*What is it?*
In this treatment either 'natural' or synthetic oestrogens are used. The most commonly used preparation is 'natural' oestrogen obtained from a pregnant mare's urine (Premarin). Some synthetic oestrogens are combined with other drugs eg. oestrogen plus progestogen  which is similar to the

contraceptive pill, given cyclically, bleeding on tablet-free days; oestrogen plus sedative where psychological symptoms (eg. insomnia) are prominent. All the above preparations are taken orally.

Implants may also be inserted under the skin under local anaesthetic and will last 6 months or a year. The main problems with implants are that if they are not suited to the patient they cannot be immediately discontinued as can tablets. They often cause unpredictable bleeding from the uterus.

## Side Effects

Nausea, breast discomfort, weight gain, bleeding. Many doctors were initially against HRT because it caused too much post-menopausal bleeding with the high doses of oestrogen used. Now it is known that much lower dosage may be used and irregular bleeding should not occur on Premarin if the dose is correctly adjusted.

Irregular bleeding is still a problem with implants and will nearly always occur in the tablet-free days of combined oestrogen/progestogen preparations as it does with the pill.

## Risks

*Clotting:*
Many doctors refuse to prescribe oestrogens for the menopause because it is now known that both the natural and synthetic oestrogens can cause clotting (hence venous thrombosis, stroke and heart attack).

*Cancer:*
There are no firm answers to this yet, as women have not been studied over long enough periods of time. But recent studies suggest that the risk of getting uterine cancer may be increased in women on HRT. The risk is related to dose and duration of therapy, so it would seem advisable to take the minimum amount necessary to control symptoms (often much less than manufacturers' recommended doses) for the shortest possible time. Some doctors believe that oestrogen plus progestogen preparations are the least likely to cause cancer. The oestrogen called stilboestrol should not be used. (see page 65)

## Who should have HRT?

Inadvisable for women with high blood pressure, high cholesterol levels, diabetes, gall bladder disease, obesity, breast, uterine or cervical cancer and for heavy smokers.

## Benefits

HRT alleviates many of the most distressing symptoms such as flushing, headaches, tiredness, irritability, loss of sex drive and vaginal discomfort.

Weighing up the possible risks and benefits is difficult, but it is clearly very much an individual matter. Hopefully, a good GP would spend a lot of time discussing the pros and cons before a joint decision is made.

## MENOPAUSE CLINICS

There are a number of these around the country; Aberdeen, Birmingham, Brighton, Bristol, Durham, Edinburgh, Glasgow, Leeds, London (King's College Hospital, Chelsea Hospital for Women), Merthyr Tydfil, Nottingham, Nuneaton, Oxford, Sheffield. Many take direct appointments as well as referrals from GPs. Some (not all) are a bit overenthusiastic about HRT.

# INFERTILITY

Infertility is certainly a physical problem to do with hormones, glands, ovulation, Fallopian tubes etc. But to the woman concerned it is also an emotional problem. We can help ourselves by knowing about the possible physical causes of infertility and by being prepared for the questions and examinations which are routine in infertility investigation/treatment situations. Sometimes we may be lucky enough to have a sympathetic doctor, who might also try to understand our emotional problems; but by talking to each other and sharing feelings about the experiences of the investigations, as well as how we are managing our lives in general, we can understand that we are far from being alone in the situation. This should help us to feel less like failures, less tense and nervous in investigatory situations, less depressed in our everyday lives.

## A FEW STATISTICS TO GET THINGS IN PERSPECTIVE

Size of problem: It is generally accepted that about 10 per cent of married couples are unable to have a child.

Share of problem: in the past, the woman has been 'blamed'. More recently, one source has it that in about half the number of cases investigated, the cause of the couple's infertility is found in the man[1]. Another source has it that, of the cases investigated, 25 per cent were due to the man's infertility, 25 per cent to the woman's, and 50 per cent were due to factors affecting them both[2]. It is said that 80 per cent of people get pregnant within one year of starting investigations.

## INITIAL INTERVIEW

The initial interview, where questions ranging from the kind of work done by the man and the woman, past illnesses and operations, menstrual history, contraceptives used, sexual techniques and marital relations etc, may (but need not, depending on the attitude and personality of the doctor) be embarrassing, but are necessary as some of the information may be suggestive of possible reasons for infertility. Knowing about our own bodies and being used to discussing psychological/sexual/marital problems with each other can really help in such situations.

## CAUSES OF INFERTILITY IN WOMEN

For systematic accounts of, reasons for, and causes of infertility, other texts should be used (see references below). Briefly, the initial examination and subsequent tests and examinations either eliminate or discover:

1) general disease which could lower fertility (eg. malfunction of one of the endocrine glands, the organs which produce hormones)
2) congenital abnormalities (eg. absence of uterus)
3) local disease of genital tract (Fallopian tubes, uterus, vagina, and vulva)
4) ovarian factors (really endocrine factors - see chapter on the Menstrual Cycle)

## TESTS AND INVESTIGATIONS

Again, for systematic accounts of reasons for the tests, and what results to expect, other texts should be read. Here is a brief summary of some of the tests carried out - their names and the procedures.

1) The woman should be asked to take her *temperature* to see if she is ovulating (see chapter on Rhythm to find out how this is done).
2) She should have her blood tested for such things as anaemia and be asked if she is taking any drugs, as some antidepressants and tranquilizers prevent ovulation.
3) The man should give a sample of sperm and be examined before any surgery is carried out on the woman. There are simple remedies for male infertility including bathing the testes in cold water (more sperms are produced in cool conditions) and Vitamin B12 injections.
4) *Post-coital or Huhner test*
This test is to check whether the man's sperm can survive in the woman's cervical mucus. The test should be carried out as near as possible to the time of ovulation (remember the effect of the changing levels of hormones throughout the menstrual cycle on the cervical mucus). The couple will be asked to have intercourse about 12-22 hours

The Post-coital Hühner test

before the woman has the test. A speculum will be inserted into her vagina, exposing her cervix, and a little of the mucus painlessly taken from it. This is examined under a microscope and the result is immediately available.
5) *Tests for tubal blockage:* There are at the moment 3 ways of testing whether the Fallopian tubes are open (patent).
   i) *Gas insufflation:* This is when carbon dioxide is blown gently, at a

certain pressure, through the uterus and tubes, from a small cylinder which has a gas-light nozzle at its tip which is inserted into the cervix. A pressure meter (a *manometer*) is attached to the cylinder, and this records the progress of the carbon dioxide. If the pressure falls, it means that the gas is passing freely through the tubes into the abdominal cavity, where it is absorbed into the blood. A stethoscope may also be used on the woman's lower abdomen; if the tubes are open, the gas can be heard passing through them.

ii) *Hysterosalpingography:* This is a special X-ray (which shows up the inside of the womb and the Fallopian tubes. (Greek words: hysteros meaning womb and salpinx meaning tube.) The test is carried out in a similar fashion to the tubal insufflation, but instead of gas, a small quantity of radio-opaque fluid (water soluble iodine) is introduced through the cervix, and outlines the cavity of the uterus and the Fallopian tubes. At suitable intervals, as the fluid passes through, X-ray photos are taken, and some X-ray departments have monitor screens on which the passage of the fluid through the uterus and Fallopian tubes can be observed as it happens. The sensation is quite like a period pain.

iii) *Laparoscopy:* This is performed under a general anaesthetic and usually involves 2 or 3 days in hospital. An instrument like a thin telescope (a *laparoscope)* is passed through a small incision (about half an inch long) which is made in the abdominal wall just below the navel. It is possible to see the contents of the pelvis clearly through the laparoscope, and, if necessary, take photographs with a special camera. To confirm that the tubes are open, blue dye is injected up through the cervix, and as it passes up through the genital tract, it can be seen coming out through the outer ends of the tubes. If the tubes are blocked an operation to clear them may be suggested. Success will depend on how badly they are damaged, the success rate out of every 100 women operated on is about 40 per cent.

6) *Endometrial Biopsy:* This test is to examine the endometrium (lining of the womb) during the second half of the menstrual cycle (remember the effect of the changing levels of hormones throughout the menstrual cycle on the endometrium) to check that:

i) the endometrium has thickened under the influence of oestrogen during the first two weeks of the cycle in readiness for the fertilized egg.

ii) progesterone is being produced by the corpus luteum (ruptured follicle) in normal quantity. Since progesterone is produced by the ovarian follicle after the follicle has ruptured, the presence of the progesterone in the blood in the second two weeks of the cycle is generally regarded as evidence that ovulation has occurred.

There are two ways of taking an endometrial biopsy. The first is known as d&c (dilatation and curettage) where, under a general anaesthetic, the lining of the womb is scraped away using a curette. The curette is a thin instrument with a rounded tip which is passed through the cervix into the uterus. The second method is where only a tiny piece of the endometrium is removed using a mini-curette, not under a general anaesthetic.

If the woman is not ovulating she may be treated by a drug called Clonid and this produces ovulation in 70 per cent of women given it. To avoid overdose (and multiple pregnancy) we suggest you go to a doctor who has a special interest in infertility and can monitor you carefully. Pergonal is another fertility drug which is difficult to regulate.

## FURTHER READING

1) *Infertility,* ed Edith Rudinger, (Consumer Association 1972)
2) *Fundamentals of Obstetrics and Gynaecology, Vol 2,* Derek Llewellyn-Jones (Faber & Faber 1972)

## ORGANIZATIONS

The National Association for the Childless and Childfree was formed to campaign for better help for couples who are having fertility problems and also to support those who have chosen not to have children. Contact National Association for the Childless and Childfree, 24B Avenue Road, London N6. Judith Lane runs a discussion group in an Oxford hospital for infertile women. Contact her at 16 James Street, Oxford.

# CONTRACEPTION

Choosing a method of birth control partly depends on its supposed efficiency. We begin our contraception section therefore with a comparative table.

| | What would happen this year to one million women who chose | No. of live births | No. of associated deaths | No. of deaths due to method | Total no. of deaths |
|---|---|---|---|---|---|
| **Age 20-24** | No birth control | 614,00 | 53 | 0 | 53 |
| | Pill | 19,000 | 2 | 13 | 15 |
| | Intra-uterine device | 19,000 | 2 | 10 | 12 |
| | Diaphragm or condom only | 160,000 | 14 | 0 | 14 |
| | Abortion only | 0 | 0 | 25 (from 1,330,000 abortions) | 25 |
| | Diaphragm or condom, plus abortion | 0 | 0 | 4 (from 206,000 abortions) | 4 |
| **Age 30-34** | No birth control | 558,000 | 100 | 0 | 100 |
| | Pill | 18,000 | 3 | 48 | 51 |
| | Intra-uterine device | 18,000 | 3 | 10 | 13 |
| | Diaphragm or condom only | 146,00 | 26 | 0 | 26 |
| | Abortion | 0 | 0 | 52 (from 1,227,000 abortions) | 52 |
| | Diaphragm or condom, plus abortion | 0 | 0 | 8 (from 196,000 abortions) | 8 |
| **Age 40-44** | No birth control | 317,000 | 183 | 0 | 183 |
| | Pill | 6,000 | 4 | 245 | 249 |
| | Intra-uterine device | 6,000 | 4 | 10 | 14 |
| | Diaphragm or condom only | 59,000 | 34 | 0 | 34 |
| | Abortion only | 0 | 0 | 66 (from 651,000 abortions) | 66 |
| | Diaphragm or condom plus abortion | 0 | 0 | 8 (from 84,000 abortions) | 8 |

# THE CAP & DIAPHRAGM

The cap is made of soft rubber, shaped like a dome and has a springy metal strip inserted in the rim. It is put up into the vagina, over the cervix, before you make love.

## FITTING

Go to your doctor (preferably at your family planning clinic as they will be trained to fit caps). There he or she will give you the right sized cap. Then, you will be shown how to put the cap in properly. Since this is very important, don't be frightened of wasting their time, or of asking silly questions. There are no silly questions in this matter, everything you don't understand is important.

Diaphragm — cap most often used

## SPERMICIDAL JELLY OR CREAM

2 ribbons (or about 1 teaspoon) of spermicidal cream or jelly must be smeared on each side of the dome of the cap, and some more spread completely around the rim, before inserting it into the vagina.

## INSERTION

A few clinics tell women to use an applicator to help insert the cap. Don't, because you can't feel what you're doing. Put the cap into your vagina, by squeezing it into an oval and sliding it back as far as it will go, the spring then regains its circular shape. Once it is in place you should be able to feel your cervix through the thin rubber.

## HOW DOES IT WORK?

Some say that the rubber barrier stops all the sperm, but we would say that the spermicidal jelly or cream sitting on the other side of the diaphragm is necessary to kill whatever sperm get around it. That is why it is so important to use a spermicide. If you make love again after 2 hours, you must put in more jelly or cream or a pessary or even use a condom. A few spermicides, (notably Rendell's Pessaries) can damage

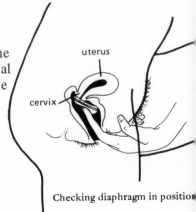

Checking diaphragm in position

36

rubber, so look out for that. Don't get too obsessional about the spermicide, thinking 'every little bit helps' covering the cap with cream. It is not necessary and might provoke allergic reaction.

## WHEN TO TAKE IT OUT

You take it out about 8 hours after intercourse, some say 6, but *never* less. In fact the longer you keep it in, the better, since it leaves more time for the semen to be killed by the cream. Don't go more than 24 hours without washing it.

When you have finished using the cap, wash and dry it but don't put talcum powder on it. Talcum powder sometimes contains strong chemicals, which could effect either you or the rubber.

## WHAT TO REMEMBER

The rubber is fragile so, before you use it, hold it up to the light to check for holes, and don't keep the same cap for more than a year.

If you lose or gain more than 7 pounds in weight, it is advisable to check with your doctor to see if you need a different sized cap.

## IS IT A GOOD METHOD?

The diaphragm, backed up with the possibility of an early abortion, is a good contraceptive. If you use it, it should be like a reflex. Every night, or morning, when you clean your teeth, you put your cap in and if you don't make love, too bad, but if you do you are safe. Some women even use it

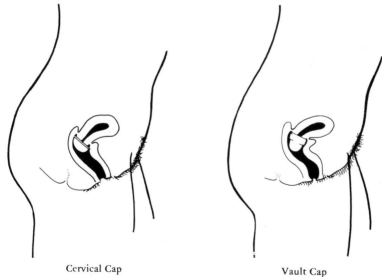

Cervical Cap                    Vault Cap

when they have their periods to collect the blood, it's less messy and cheaper than buying tampons.

In fact, it's a good way of getting confidence in your ability to cope with your body. It's a contraceptive where you have to be active, to overcome prejudices. Men might also learn how to fit a cap in their partners or help them. That would mean a change for them, for us, for everybody, wouldn't it?

Since first writing this chapter women have told us they also use cervical and vault caps which sit directly onto the cervix. If your muscles are too slack to have a diaphragm it might be worth asking if it's possible to be fitted with one of these.

# SPERMICIDES

Spermicides are chemical contraceptives sold mainly over the counter or through mail order, though clinics and doctors give them out too. There are 3 forms: creams which come in tubes, foams in aerosol containers, or tablets and pessaries—vaginal suppositories.

A woman has to put a spermicide up into her vagina before intercourse. The product having filled the vagina, its chemical property will kill sperms before they reach the uterus. In theory that is absolutely true—spermicides once in contact with sperms kill them, but a product is always tested under laboratory conditions, which is to say in a dish where a spermicide cannot miss sperms. In practice this is only half the story. In the vaginal setting, it is quite easy for some sperm to escape from the spermicide. A lot of precautions must be observed for the proper functioning of spermicides and too often the manufacturers either 'forget' them or else mention them in a very misleading way. It seems that as long as they can fulfil the laboratory tests, manufacturers can do what they like in terms of the way they market the product. As the marketing report of one such manufacturer put it 'as long as the product is effective and usable, what the customer does is not the concern of the manufacturer'.

This is one type of foam applicator

Here now are the conditions that the user has to observe:

1) A spermicide MUST NEVER BE USED ALONE. Many women followed false statements like the one given with Rendell's Pessaries that claimed 'no further precautions need be taken' and they got pregnant. Alarmed by this, the Family Planning Association (FPA) advises now that spermicides should always be used with a cap or a sheath.

2) A spermicide must be inserted very high in the vagina, and as some women have very short fingers and a long vagina, they cannot reach the cervix. It must be inserted 20 minutes to 1 hour before intercourse, and if ejaculation has not occurred within this time a reinsertion is recommended. Here again there may be misinformation by the manufacturers, since they suggest allowing 'an hour before' as the deadline, but an hour before what?

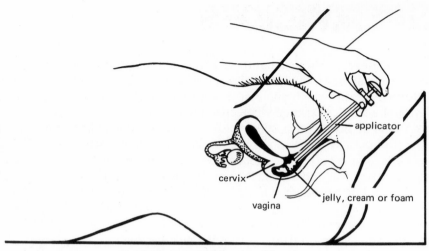

Putting in spermicidal cream with an inserter

3) If too old the spermicide loses its properties and no longer kills sperm; foaming tablets and pessaries will deteriorate quickly if kept in hot or damp places. Tablets should be checked, and if they do not foam, thrown away. Not one product bears a date stamp ...

4) With repeated use some spermicides damage rubber so if you are using a cap make sure that your spermicide isn't one of them.

5) Some women can react to spermicides; reactions include rashes, itching, burning and cystitis. Although the problem can usually be solved by change of brand, the symptoms are similar to those of vaginal infection and sometimes doctors may treat them as such.

6) Douching and bathing should be avoided immediately after intercourse.

It would have been too tedious to mention all the misleading information which make spermicides quite unreliable, and explain the high rate of failures of this method of contraception when used alone. Nevertheless bearing in mind all the conditions under which spermicides must be used they can be quite useful. The next step is to get the manufacturers to give correct information.

# THE SHEATH

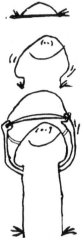

The sheath is a method of contraception used by men. It is unrolled on to the erect penis to contain the sperm before any of them can be released into the woman's vagina. It is safest when used with a spermicide; then if the condom bursts or comes off, the result is less likely to be disastrous.

There are three types of sheath:

1) teat ended: they have a space for the semen.

2) plain ended: you must leave a space for the semen

3) shaped: they are bulbous just behind the teat and are said to fit more comfortably over the tip of the penis.

Many of the brands are lubricated, which is helpful if the vagina is dry.

## IMPORTANT THINGS TO REMEMBER

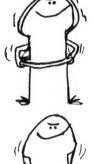

The tip of the condom should be squeezed as it is put on, to leave the teat (or about half an inch at the end if it does not have a teat) empty of air. Otherwise the air between the sheath and the penis could make the rubber tear.

After his orgasm, the man must withdraw immediately since the sheath can easily slip off if you carry on moving. This must be done very carefully, holding the sheath in place with the fingers.

Never use a sheath more than once, unless you buy a re-usable washable sheath (its thick rubber makes it quite a drag). Used very often, condoms are quite expensive: 30p on average for three. However since it is sold over the counter, it's still the most widely used contraceptive in England.

We asked a man friend of ours what it was like to use a condom. What he said was that it was a drag to put on, one has to be sexually confident, one can't have a 'nice rest inside', there is loss of feeling . . .

We don't pretend that the condom is the most marvellous contraceptive. However it can be quite useful.

# INTRA-UTERINE DEVICES

An intra-uterine device is a small, flexible object made of plastic, plastic and copper, or (rarely these days) stainless steel. It is inserted through the opening in the cervix into the uterus.

The more common types in use nowadays are:

1) Copper Seven for women who have not had a full term pregnancy, or Copper T, similar to the Copper Seven but T-shaped. This kind of IUD has one thin black string.

2) Lippes Loop has two strings of different colours according to size and is for women who have had one or more children.

3) Safe-T Coil has two green strings. This is also for women who have had children.

4) Dalkon Shield has one thick black string. NO ONE SHOULD HAVE THIS KIND; the shape will tell you why. It has been withdrawn in the USA and is not recommended by the FPA in this country. If you have a Dalkon Shield you should have it out with a local anaesthetic as you may need to be dilated in order to remove it. If you were not told what kind of IUD you were having at the time of insertion you should be able to tell by the strings.

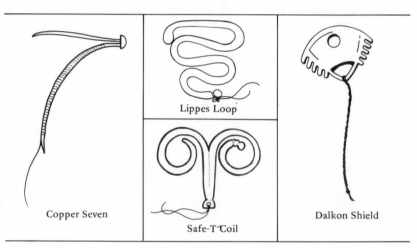

Copper Seven

Lippes Loop

Safe-T Coil

Dalkon Shield

## HOW DOES IT WORK?

There are many theories as to how the IUD works. It certainly disturbs and irritates the inside of your uterus (hence the increased discharge some women have) and often infects it. One study by W L Faulkner and H W Ory in the *Journal of the American Medical Association* 1976, no. 235 suggests that IUD users run five times the risk of contracting pelvic infection than non-users. We are concerned that many women with IUDs get pregnant while taking antibiotics or aspirin for some other problem. We believe that this happens because the effect of the IUD has been cancelled out and we urge women to use some other form of contraception as well while taking these drugs.

## INSERTION

The effectiveness rate gets higher and the complications rate lower when the device is inserted by a trained person; most GPs are not trained to fit IUDs and if you don't know about yours, you'll be better off going to an FPA clinic.

It is best to have it done while you are having a period because when you menstruate the os, the entrance to the uterus, is a little bigger, making the insertion easier; also you know you are not pregnant which is very important. Unfortunately the insertion can be painful so it is best not to plan to do anything else that day. You may have no reaction at all, you may need to rest for a few minutes or feel quite wobbly afterwards and have to take a taxi home. Very occasionally, some women get a kind of shock and their blood pressure drops. This is why medical back-up is important. It is best to take a friend.

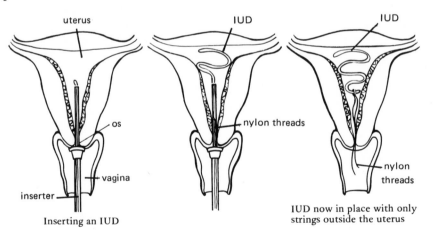

Inserting an IUD

IUD now in place with only strings outside the uterus

## FOLLOW UP

Check after each period if the thread
is still there, by feeling for it or
by looking with a speculum. It
will look like this.

## REMOVAL

To remove an IUD someone just has to
pull on the string and it will come out.
A self help group can remove them
except for Dalkon Shields. No one
knows how long an IUD should be
kept in. One thing that might happen
is that secretions may get calcified on
the coil so it will get coated. This happens
with the Copper Seven so doctors say it is
advisable to change a Copper Seven every 3 years. With the other kinds of
IUD, as long as you are happy with it, why worry?

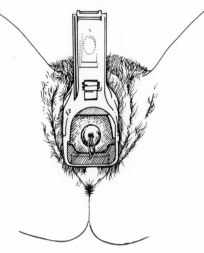

View of os with speculum in place—
IUD strings showing

## EXPLUSION

8 to 10 per cent of women find their IUDs self-expelled in one year. If it
comes out or you can no longer feel or see the thread go back to the clinic.

## SIDE EFFECTS AND COMPLICATIONS

1) Because there is a foreign body in the uterus periods are often heavier
and last longer, although this often settles down.

2) You might feel some backache and cramps after insertion. This is
the uterus trying to expel the device, rather like the discomfort when the
eyes are getting used to contact lenses.

3) Irregular bleeding, irritation or smelly discharge indicates a heavy
infection. This may mean that you should have the IUD removed. Infection
can spread from the uterus to the Fallopian tubes (salpingitis). Salpingitis
jeopardizes your chances of child-bearing because it blocks the Fallopian
tubes, so an egg cannot pass. The infection can spread into the abdomen
(pelvic inflammatory disease). This is very serious.

4) On rare occasions, the device can perforate the uterus or embed itself in the wall.

# WHO SHOULD NOT USE AN IUD

1) Women with a recent or current infection of the uterus or Fallopian tubes.

2) Immediately after a Caesarian section.

3) Women with cysts, fibroids or erosion of the cervix.

4) Women who might be pregnant.

5) In the first 6 weeks following abortion or childbirth, as it would be hard to distinguish what was causing any complication.

There is a new kind of IUD which may become available to British women. It is T-shaped and contains progesterone which is gradually released into the uterine cavity over a long period—1 or 3 years depending on which model. The progesterone makes the mucus in the cervical canal thick and dry, preventing sperm from entering. It also probably affects the endometrium. It might be a good way to bypass the depression some women get from taking progesterone orally but the disadvantage of this method would be that the device would need changing and it is a little harder to insert than other IUDs.

Doctors describe the most suitable women for the IUD as being 'feckless and fertile' and 'too stupid to use anything else'. This usually means unsupported mothers, poor women with lots of kids and so on. These women are very often not medically suitable for the IUD. They may be anaemic from a poor diet and cannot afford to lose more blood from heavy periods. They may have an undiagnosed uterine infection made much worse by an IUD. We must guard against being stereotyped and fight to make our own fully informed decisions..

# THE PILL

## THE COMBINED PILL

### How Does it Work?

On the fifth day after a period begins you take the first pill and continue taking one pill a day until the pack is finished. The 'combined' pill consists of two synthetic substances which are similar to the natural hormones—oestrogen and progesterone—which the body produces.

*Oestrogen:*
The oestrogen in the pill is just enough to prevent the pituitary gland from sending out its usual message (FSH) for an egg to develop. By taking oestrogen every day for 20, 21 or 22 days (depending on the type of pill you have) you avoid having an egg develop at all that month. Your ovaries remain inactive. There is thus no egg to be fertilized by the sperm.

*Progestogen:*
A little progestogen every day provides two vital back up effects:

1) it keeps the mucus plug in the cervix thick and dry, so sperm have a hard time getting through

2) it keeps the lining of the uterus from developing properly, so if an egg does ripen (if the oestrogen level of the pill is too low for you) or if you forget a pill and the sperm gets through the cervical mucus and fertilizes the egg, the fertilized egg will not be able to find a good place on the lining to implant.

When you have stopped taking your course of pills, the sudden drop in oestrogen and progestogen makes the lining of the uterus start to disintegrate. On about day 28 you have your 'pill period' which will probably be lighter than usual because of the effect of the progestogen in the Pill.

There are many different kinds of combined pill. Most women are on pills with low dosages of oestrogen (ie 50 micrograms or less) in order to minimize the risk of thrombosis. There are pills with no oestrogen in them at all; but these progestogen-only pills (described below) are less effective as they do not prevent ovulation.

*Low dose pills (50 micrograms of oestrogen—0.05 mg):*
Some of these, for example Ovran and Eugynon 50, contain, as the progestogen, 0.5 mg di-norgestrol. This is a powerful progestogen and therefore not as much is needed as with other progestogens. However it is not known if this increased potency offsets the advantages of low-dose oestrogen pill. Only long term follow up and research will answer this question.

Other low dose pills, eg Demulen 50 or Gynovlar, contain varying amounts of different types of progestogen. It is possible in pills containing progestogen such as norgestrol, for the oestrogen content to be reduced still further. This is because these progestogens themselves have 'oestrogenic activity'.

*Extra low dose pills:*
eg. Eugynon 30, Microgynon 30, Ovranette contain 30 micrograms (0.03mg) of oestrogen, and norgestrol. Loestrin 20 contains 0.02mg oestrogen and 1 mg of progestogen (not norgestrol). The makers say that Loestrin cuts out many of the side effects created by other pills. However, it is thought to be a less effective contraceptive.

Different pills react on different women in different ways. If one pill suits one woman, it will not necessarily suit you. Similarly, if the first pill you try does not suit you, it is possible that the next pill will ... at least for a bit (see Side Effects).

## WHAT YOUR DOCTOR SHOULD DO

She/he should take a detailed case history to find out if there is any record for example of high blood pressure during pregnancy, diabetes etc. She/he should then do a careful physical examination including breasts, pelvic examination etc, not just a smear test. Some doctors take urine samples to test for abnormal amounts of sugar in the urine which can be due to diabetes.

*You should be told to look out for and report symptoms such as:* headaches; sudden or severe complete or partial loss of vision, seeing 'stars', severe leg or chest pains or unexplained cough. You should stop taking the pill and report these immediately. You should also be told to report irregular or missed periods.

*You should be monitored closely if you have or develop any of the following:* heart or kidney disease, asthma, high blood pressure, epilepsy, fibroids in the womb, diabetes and hepatitis or liver disease.

*In any case, the following should be checked regularly:* blood pressure, breasts, pelvic examination, cervical smear taken, any migraine or depressive features. Blood and urine tests are also often necessary, particularly for older women.

*The older you are* the more important it is that you should be monitored carefully, as there is little experience of long term use on women from 45 years upwards on the Pill. A leader article in the *BMJ* (8.6.74) suggests that tests for phlebitis, glucose tolerance and liver function might also be necessary.

# EFFICACY

The Pill, if taken as directed, is virtually 100 per cent effective in preventing conception. (The more strongly progestogenic pills such as Gynovlar or Anovlar have a larger safety margin if a tablet is missed. If you are over-weight, you might require larger doses of both hormones for effectiveness.) Because it is so effective, and because it has the backing of many influential people throughout the world it is widely used.

*The Pill does very occasionally fail to prevent conception,* and doctors have often explained these failures by saying that they must have been due to the woman's forgetfulness or stupidity. However, such doctors have now been shown to be as fallible as ever. Firstly it has become clear that an upset stomach causing vomiting or diarrhoea can prevent the Pill from being absorbed: if you do experience vomiting or diarrhoea, particularly early on in your cycle, you may be wise to take extra pre-cautions for the rest of the month, and/or to take an extra pill.

Secondly, the Pill's functioning can be affected by other drugs. So far, Rifampicin (an antibiotic for the treatment of TB) has been shown to do this, and some other antibiotics, analgesics such as aspirin and phenacetin, and the anti-epileptic drugs are suspected too. Given the Pill's low failure rate, this might not be as serious as it sounds. However, it is likely that as the drugs in the Pill are reduced in quantity there will be correspondingly more likelihood of its being rendered ineffective when taken with other drugs. It is wise, therefore, if taking other drugs, to be alert to a missed period or any breakthrough bleeding and if you are paranoid about getting pregnant, to use another form of contraception. If a pill is missed you can take it up to 12 hours late and still be protected. Otherwise another method may be needed until the next package is started. If you forget a pill for over 12 hours, you could actually trigger ovulation by taking another pill, depending on which kind of pill you are using. Read the instructions on the packet of *your* pills: some say take a double dose for the following 2 days; others say that you should just carry on as normal—in which case you may run the risk of getting pregnant even until the first 2 weeks of your next cycle.

For the first 2 weeks on the Pill—some say for the first cycle—other pre-cautions are necessary. It is also sometimes advised that other precautions should be taken for one month if you change to another brand, particularly if it is of a lower dosage.

## IF THE PILL FAILS

If you do become pregnant while taking it, you are unlikely to find out for some time, with the result that abortion would not be by the simplest method and may be out of the question altogether. (As the Pill can have teratogenic effects, ie.effects on the foetus—there are strong reasons for having an abortion.) Most babies born following Pill failure appear to be normal but possible latent effects are unknown and are not being systematically studied.

## IS THE PILL SAFE?

Recent propaganda would have us believe that this is the case. A large scale study by the Royal College of General Practitioners was widely reported as giving the pill a 'clean bill of health' and other such eulogies. The facts in the study did not however point to that conclusion and it is very difficult to see how the study's main conclusions were reached. (For an analysis of the study and its bias, see 'Information or Propaganda', *Spare Rib* 32.)

There is no easy answer to 'Is the Pill safe?'. It depends who you are, where you live, how old you are, your family and medical histories, the competence of your doctor, whether you are a heavy smoker to name but a few relevant factors. It might seem reassuring to learn that the overall risk of death from thrombosis as a result of pregnancy is 20 times greater than that from the Pill. Statistics like this have always been used to 'show' that the Pill is safe, but this is a misuse of statistics. As I have said earlier, there are so many relevant factors concerning each individual that one cannot make a decision based on generalizations. Furthermore, while the pill may be an efficient alternative to pregnancy, it is not the only one. There are also many unanswered questions and much that is not understood about the Pill. Sometimes the right questions are not being asked, or research fundings are mysteriously stopped, as in the case in the USA with research on the Pill for possible connections with cervical cancer and diabetes[1]. The most obvious question to which there is as yet no answer is the question of long term effects. While there is no proof that it causes cancer for example, the effect on a woman taking the pill for the majority of her child-bearing years has not been ascertained. Some people fear that middle-aged women who were long term users may be more at risk to vascular diseases, heart attacks and diabetes.

The truth is that even if there are no obvious reasons why we should not take the Pill, we cannot make a truly informed decision. The Pill is still, to some degree, an experiment, although you would never get that impression from the 'information' we are given. The scandalous way in which the American FDA approved the first pill on the basis of a study of only 132 women 'volunteers' is still being perpetuated to some extent today. (Among that group of women there were two who died of severe chest pain and an autopsy was not performed on either of them.) The FDA has no records of their deaths[2].

Sometimes the experts compare the safety of the Pill and its inducement of an artificially pregnant state with that of a natural pregnancy. Such people, far from being experts in the field of pharmacology are usually only gynaecologists with very little training in pharmacology. Contrary to what their names imply, the substances in the pill are synthetic, not natural. Women and doctors are thus misled by this false labelling. Harold Speert, an American gynaecologist, feels that to give a true impression the substances should have been given chemical names (like those they use in the petroleum industry)[3].

## WHAT IS KNOWN TO DATE?

It is impossible to provide comprehensive information in so small a space, and in any case, new discoveries are being made all the time. However, listed below are the most important facts. For more detailed information, consult *Our Bodies, Ourselves* (see Further Reading).

**The Following Women Would be Best Advised Not to Take the Pill:**

1) Women over 40, because of the increased risk of heart attack; likewise women over 35 who have other risk factors (eg. diabetes, obesity, heavy smoking, high blood pressure) should also not take the Pill for the same reason. However, although the American FDA has issued a nationwide recommendation concerning women over 40, it has not done the same for the latter group. The most serious side effects tend to appear in women over 35 particularly if they smoke heavily, are overweight or immobile. (For a fuller explanation see *Women's Report* 3/5.)

2) Women with breast cancer or certain other cancers, serious liver disease or vaginal bleeding of unknown cause.

3) Women with 'Sickle-cell' anaemia (a form of anaemia which Negro women can have). Black women should be tested for this.

4) Women conditions to do with poor blood circulation, eg. clotting, bad varicose veins.

IF YOU HAVE OR DEVELOP THE FOLLOWING and decide to take the Pill you should be monitored closely (some specialists might think you should not take it—it will depend on other relevant factors like age etc): family history of breast or uterine cancer, diabetes, migraine, epilepsy, asthma, mild varicose veins, high blood pressure, tendency to severe depression.

## SIDE EFFECTS

It is becoming clear that all tissues and organs are affected by the Pill in some way. Side effects are bound to occur, some being welcome and some being unwelcome and possibly dangerous. There is now a long list of known possible side effects, the list is still growing; (for a relatively comprehensive list see reference 3).

Some side effects such as unexpected vaginal bleeding, breast tenderness, weight gain and nausea disappear after the first 3 months. If any side effects persist they should be reported to your doctor. Side effects can however, suddenly appear after some time on the pill even as long as 10 years. So far evidence suggests that the body reverts to normal when you stop taking it. Most changes are reversed after short periods on the Pill, but we don't yet know about long periods. Apparently the majority of women on the pill notice no troublesome side effects, but some women can be very much affected by them in ways such as the following:

## Mood Changes

Contrary to what some studies purport to show it is undoubtedly true that the Pill can affect mood, ranging from mild to severe depression, libido changes, irritability and other pre-menstrual type symptoms. Depression can be difficult to spot because it can happen gradually. Friends who notice changes can be useful here. Many women who stop the Pill following remarks from friends experience 'feeling themselves' or 'a great weight taken off their backs'. Some people think that the leading cause of death from the Pill is suicide from the depression and not thrombosis (*B J Psych*, Lewis and Hoghughi). With mood changes and headaches (see below) the highest incidences appear to be in pills with higher doses of progestogen and low doses of oestrogen (*British Medical Journal (BMJ)*, 28.9.68). These particular pills appear to induce in the woman a state similar to the normal pre-menstrual phase, the difference being that the pill-induced phase lasts nearly three weeks. Thus the new pills with low doses of oestrogen can be a mixed blessing to some women. This serves to illustrate how Pill 'developments' can be one step back as well as one step forward: most brands of Pill now in use are of this high progestogen/low oestrogen variety. Some women who develop depression can be helped by Vitamin B6, but it depends on whether they have a B6 deficiency or not and, if so, of what kind (*Lancet* 31.8.74 p 516).

## Headaches and Migraine

It is well known that changes in hormone balance (eg. during the normal menstrual cycle, during pregnancy) can affect the incidence of headaches or migraine. However, in spite of this, the RCGP study attempted to show that the increased incidence in these symptoms 'could be entirely due to (patient) bias'! There appear to be more Pill-taking headache and migraine sufferers among the younger age-groups than in non Pill-taking women (see *Migraine News* March 1974). The Pill can have a beneficial effect on previous migraine sufferers but this, according to Dr Ellen Grant, tends to wear off so that migraines eventually become more frequent. She has found that headaches tended to improve if the Pill was stopped, but in a few cases they were exacerbated (*BMJ* 17.8.68). If migraine occurs at the end of the Pill cycle, continuous Pill taking can often get rid of the symptoms.

## Dosage and Tolerance

'It is possible to produce mood and vascular (ie. blood vessel) reactions in everyone by altering their hormone balance although there is a wide variation in tolerance to these effects and the time they take to develop' (Dr Grant). It has also been found that women who react dramatically to normal hormone changes such as pregnancy or menstruation appear to react most quickly to the Pill no matter what the dose or type, while the least reactive 'have no overt symptoms for as long as 10 years' (Dr Grant). In other words, if at first your body appears to tolerate the Pill, it is possible that in time symptoms might appear. By varying the dosage, symptoms *can* be cleared up, but Dr Grant has found the same problem as with the introduction of the low oestrogen Pill: in 'reactive' women, she found that by curing one symptom, another one would develop (eg. depression, irregular bleeding, vein complaints). She found that pill takers reactive to headaches and other blood vessel complaints seem to be more susceptible to other symptoms such as mood changes and weight gain.

## Implications

Some women will feel that seemingly non-life threatening symptoms such as those described above are a small price to pay for relief from worries of pregnancy, but it is worth bearing in mind that blood vessel changes in one part of the body may parallel changes in vessels in other parts of the body. While some blood vessel changes, such as headaches can be tolerable, others could be dangerous. (See Dr Grant, above.)

## More Dangerous Blood Vessel Reactions

Oedema (swelling), phlebitis (inflamation, thrombosis (blood-clotting).
The most serious of these is thrombosis. It can occur anywhere. If it occurs in the heart (*myocardial infarction*) or a major artery (*coronary thrombosis*), it is extremely dangerous. The clot (*thrombus*) can become detached and travel to a major organ, thus becoming a thromboembolism. *Pulmonary embolism* means a clot travelling to the lung; strokes involve clots travelling to the brain (strokes can also be caused by bleeding inside the brain). Clots formed in the bigger veins eg. deep vein thrombosis of the leg are more dangerous than in the smaller ones. While many women experience no such problems on the Pill it is true that among Pill takers the risk of developing a clot is increased between 5 and 6 times over. The mortality rate from clotting is similarly increased, although of course it is still relatively small (c.3 per 100,000 users). Clotting is a serious matter and even if death is avoided, the blood circulation can be permanently affected. Out of between 1,200 and 2,000 Pill users, one will be hospital-

ized. (NB the older you are the bigger the risk of clotting—either from pregnancy or from the Pill. The risks quoted above are averaged out between *all* women, regardless of other risk factors, such as weight or age.)

## Heart Attacks (Coronary Thrombosis)

All women on the Pill appear to run a 3-5 fold higher risk of heart attack than other women. The risk seems to be higher for women with certain predisposing risk factors; heavy smoking, obesity, diabetes, high blood pressure and age (over 40). The length of time a woman is on the Pill also appears to increase the risk. In women over 30, the risk of heart attack is greater than that for clotting.

## Hypertension (High Blood Pressure)

The Pill causes increases in blood pressure in some women. High blood pressure in itself increases susceptibility to severe problems such as stroke. The incidence of hypertension appears to increase with age, weight and increased duration of Pill use.

## Breasts

While it is not yet proved whether the Pill can or cannot cause breast cancer, it is now being widely stated that the Pill has a beneficial effect on the breasts as concluded in the RCGP report. However, this conclusion does not appear to be valid (see *Spare Rib* no 32). A more recent study (published in the *Lancet* 26.5.75) has been hailed as 'reassuring'. Again, this study needs to be seen in perspective: only 14 percent of the women studied had used the Pill for more than 2 years. The reassuring reports that pill-takers experience a lower incidence of benign breast growths than other women must be balanced against the experience of specialists in breast diseases. Ian Burn of Charing Cross Hospital reports for example that certain women are hypersensitive as far as their breasts are concerned to components in the Pill. 'I see many such women in my clinic every week

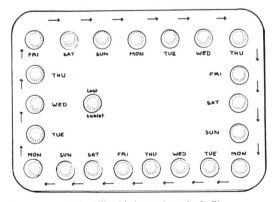

The Pill—this is one brand of pill

and in some cases it is necessary to remove the lumps concerned. In most instances, however, the lumps disappear when the "pill" is discontinued'. (personal communication).

### Effect on Fertility

There appears to be a *slightly* higher chance of being infertile after taking the Pill. The first study to investigate the Pill's effect on fertility[4] found that in women who had never had a child, significantly fewer women successfully conceived within a certain period of time after they had come off the Pill than a similar group of non-Pill takers.

### Effects on Offspring

Babies conceived by women while they are on the Pill are not being systematically studied at present, so effects on offspring are for the time being unknown. There is not, however, any discernable effect as yet. Women who stop the Pill because they wish to conceive are advised to wait for a few cycles for it has been shown that offspring conceived immediately after the mother has ceased taking the Pill are more likely to be abnormal. (*Women's Report* 3/4.) Babies who are breastfed while their mothers are on the Pill have also not been studied.

## PROGESTOGEN ONLY PILL

Examples: Femulen, Micronor and Noriday. The progestogen-only Pill is slightly less effective than the combined Pill, particularly if it is not taken as directed. Thus it is very important to follow the instructions. These are, to start on the first day of the menstrual period and to take it *at the same time* every day, continuously, without a break.

Even though the majority of users of these pills have breakthrough bleeding, and depression and blood sugar problems remain, there are thought to be no clotting or high blood pressure risks as there are with oestrogen. Unlike the combined Pill, the progestogen-only Pill does not appear to prevent *ectopic* (outside the womb) pregnancies.

## HOW DO YOU DECIDE WHETHER TO TAKE THE PILL?

Ultimately, it is *your* decision. It's not a very easy or pleasant decision to have to make. There is bound to be a lot of pressure, not least from doctors who think they know best. As I have tried to show, they don't necessarily know best and they might know a good deal less than you. Undoubtedly many women will feel forced to take the Pill because if they used another method, they could not rely on abortion facilities. This only serves to show how politics enters into the most personal parts of our lives. Whatever choice you make, you are not able to make a free one.

Women will only be able to make such a choice when we have come together and won the fight for free, safe contraception and abortion for all. Only then can we hope to rid ourselves of the constant fear of either unwanted pregnancy or of long term effects from man-made, man-invented contraceptives.

## REFERENCES

1 *Ms magazine* June 1975

2 *The Pill on Trial,* Paul Vaughan (Penguin 1972): dispassionate account of the way the Pill was developed: poses more questions than it answers.

3 *Questions and Answers* about the Pill compiled by a group of women, available from Sue Barlow, 150 Moselle Ave, London N22. (send s.a.e.)

4 'Long-term follow-up study of women using different methods of contraception—an interim report', *Journal of Biosocial Science 8,* 1976 p 373.

## FURTHER READING

*Our Bodies, Ourselves,* ed Angela Phillips and Jill Rakusen, (Penguin 1978)

# DEPO-PROVERA (D-P)

Depo—provera is an injectable contraceptive which lasts for 3 or 6 months. D—P is being used on an increasing scale in some 70 countries including Britain. It is manufactured in the US, and exported on a large scale, mostly to underdeveloped countries. But it is not licensed for use in America, and in Britain the Committee on Safety of Medicines (CSM) has only approved it for short-term use.

The US Food and Drug Administration banned the oral form of D—P in 1971 after it was found that it could cause breast cancer in beagles. The injectable form was refused a licence when there was found to be double the expected incidence of cervical cancer in women using the drug. Yet the UN Children's Fund, the World Health Organization and the International Planned Parenthood Federation all distribute D—P.

The drug contains a progestogen derived from the same source as two other progestogens which have been implicated in breast cancer studies similar to those carried out on D—P, and which were recently withdrawn. There is also a suspicion that it may cause permanent damage to the pituitary/adrenal system which has potentially very serious consequences; other types of hormonal contraception, such as the Pill, are not suspicious in this way.

The drug can produce disturbing side effects, and studies have shown that these have caused high percentages of women (25 per cent or more) to stop using it. The possibility of infertility has also been shown to exist, and in some countries the drug is restricted to women with completed families. But in Thailand, for example, it is being given to more and more young women. Little if any work has been done on the effects of D—P on offspring.

Although the CSM has as yet withheld full approval, doctors are entitled to use D—P in whatever way they wish. In a recent article in *General Practitioner*, Dr David Delvin reports how disregard of the CSM's guidelines is widespread. Throughout the country hundreds of women are being given D—P, and a number of doctors have started using it on a longer-term basis—'mainly for women who are at their wits' end to find something that will stop them getting pregnant.' Given what is known—or rather what is not known—about this experimental drug, it is not to be recommended, particularly for women who might consider having children in the future.

## FURTHER READING

1) 'Depo-provera: Third World Women Not Told This Contraceptive is on Trial', Jill Rakusen, *Spare Rib* 42, p 22

2) 'Depo—provera: Still for Sale', Jill Rakusen, *Spare Rib* 47, p 26

# RHYTHM

Recently there has been a renewal of interest in the rhythm method because many women are made miserable and ill by contraceptives – the coil and the Pill in particular. Many women using the rhythm method also use a barrier contraceptive, such as a diaphragm or sheath, and foam, to increase effectiveness. It is essential to keep records for a long time (most books recommend one year) before you can rely on knowing when you ovulate. Use several of the following methods to find this out.

## OBSERVING SIGNS

There are lucky women who get very noticeable signs that they are ovulating: some get a cramp as the egg leaves the ovary; others experience a big change in emotional and sexual feelings at that time. We can also learn to tell when we are ovulating by self examination. Sometimes the os widens a little and very often we can see a secretion leaving the os that is transparent and sticky like raw egg white. Under a microscope, ovulation secretion shows fern-like shapes and self help groups can use this method to find when they are ovulating.

## CALCULATING OVULATION TIME

The egg lives for about 12 hours and sperm for 48-72 hours in the Fallopian tubes, so you must avoid intercourse for 5 days before ovulation and 1 day after. However long your cycle is, you probably ovulate 12-16 days before

| Length of Shortest Period | First unsafe day after start of any period. | Length of Longest Period | Last unsafe day after start of any period. |
|---|---|---|---|
| 21 DAYS | 3rd DAY | 21 DAYS | 10th DAY |
| 22 DAYS | 4th DAY | 22 DAYS | 11th DAY |
| 23 DAYS | 5th DAY | 23 DAYS | 12th DAY |
| 24 DAYS | 6th DAY | 24 DAYS | 13th DAY |
| 25 DAYS | 7th DAY | 25 DAYS | 14th DAY |
| 26 DAYS | 8th DAY | 26 DAYS | 15th DAY |
| 27 DAYS | 9th DAY | 27 DAYS | 16th DAY |
| 28 DAYS | 10th DAY | 28 DAYS | 17th DAY |
| 29 DAYS | 11th DAY | 29 DAYS | 18th DAY |
| 30 DAYS | 12th DAY | 30 DAYS | 19th DAY |
| 31 DAYS | 13th DAY | 31 DAYS | 20th DAY |
| 32 DAYS | 14th DAY | 32 DAYS | 21st DAY |
| 33 DAYS | 15th DAY | 33 DAYS | 22nd DAY |
| 34 DAYS | 16th DAY | 34 DAYS | 23rd DAY |
| 35 DAYS | 17th DAY | 35 DAYS | 24th DAY |
| 36 DAYS | 18th DAY | 36 DAYS | 25th DAY |
| 37 DAYS | 19th DAY | 37 DAYS | 26th DAY |
| 38 DAYS | 20th DAY | 38 DAYS | 27th DAY |

How to calculate the 'safe' and 'unsafe' days

your next period, so forget about 'the dangerous time in the middle'. Write down the first day of your period as day 1, and the day before your next period as the last day of your cycle. At the end of 12 cycles, count up the number of days in the shortest and longest ones. Subtract 18 from the shortest cycle's number. This will give you the first unsafe day. Subtract 11 from the longest cycle's number. This will give you the last unsafe day. Go on recording your cycles each month and calculate from the last 12.

## TEMPERATURE CHARTS

This method involves taking your temperature first thing every morning before you get up or have a drink, and charting the slight changes that occur during a woman's cycle. After each period the temperature is low, dropping lower on ovulation, rising afterwards and staying up until the next period. You need to get charts and a special thermometer which will register the slight changes, as well as leaflets and advice from a clinic. Below is one woman's temperature chart.

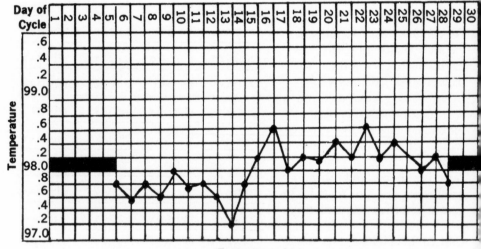

Temperature chart

If you are interested in using the rhythm method plus astrological charts, get *Natural Birth Control* by Art Rosenblum (Aquarius 1973) for instructions on working out fertility periods.

Some of us feel that if a woman lives an ordered, calm life from month to month, this method will work. But how many women live like that?

# STERILIZATION

Making a thoughtful, personal decision to have either no children or no more, and therefore asking for and obtaining a sterilization, is not as straightforward as it should be. Many women ask and are refused, on the grounds that they may regret the decision later. The operation has to be regarded as irreversible, so total confidence in this as a right process for you is of great importance. Doctors also seem often to make a moral judgment that a woman unable to procreate is one about to launch into sexual promiscuity, and the approval and consent of a husband, where there is one, is always sought. This is not a legal requirement, though people may try to make you feel it is.

Acceptable medical grounds for sterilization are: having a large number of children; the risk that another pregnancy would damage your heaith; inability to tolerate the coil and the Pill. Social grounds include: a previous abortion – proof of determination not to have children; not wanting to spend the next 20 years on the Pill. The more articulate and intelligent you sound, the more assured you are of success. One golden rule is not to be emotional and say, 'If I get pregnant again I'll kill myself'; if you seem to be unstable, they will think you are likely to change your mind about sterilization after it is too late. You must present a decisive, rational argument.

Several of the charitable pregnancy advisory services offer sterilization to both females and males. The cost is currently about £85 for a woman and £30 for a man. (If you are a monogamous couple, and likely to stay that way, vasectomy would be a good idea as it is a much simpler operation.)

Many women are pressured into sterilization as a condition of an NHS abortion. This is not the best time to make such a decision; nor is the time immediately after childbirth. Although it might seem a good idea to get everything over in one go, there is evidence of an increased mortality rate when these two operations are combined. More than one third of the NHS abortions carried out in 1973 included sterilization.

The traditional method of sterilization is called tubal ligation and requires general anaesthesia and a fairly large abdominal incision. A piece of each Fallopian tube is cut out and the two ends are tied and folded back into the surrounding tissue. Some doctors, particularly when they are doing an abortion as well, tie the tubes through a small incision at the back of the upper vagina.

The after-effects are the usual ones that follow a general anaesthetic, soreness, and some pain from the abdominal wound. A hospital stay of 8-10 days is necessary.

There is a newer operation available in some parts of the country, known as laparoscopy and tubal diathermy. Some doctors think that it can be

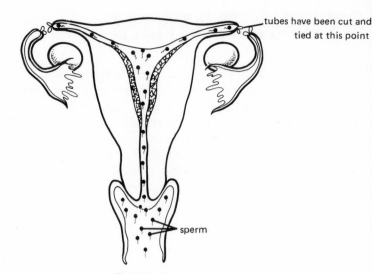

tubes have been cut and
tied at this point

sperm

Tubal ligation

performed on an out-patient basis, while others think it is too dangerous to be carried out at all. With this method, a laparoscope, which is a tiny, thin tube with mirrors and lights, is inserted into the abdomen through a ½ inch incision. The tubes are visually located and sealed up by heating (cauterization) with a small instrument inserted through another ½ inch incision. This procedure necessitates a 2-3 day stay in hospital, less discomfort than with tube-tying, and of course less scarring. One problem is that a doctor not used to doing laparoscopies cannot be sure that what he is cauterizing is in fact the tube. Some women say you should either go to somewhere like British Pregnancy Advisory Service (BPAS), where they are used to doing this operation, or else make sure beforehand that you are going to have an experienced doctor! Take a friend with you if you are going to ask questions about this.

Sterilization does not bring on early menopause, or menopausal symptoms. The menstrual cycle continues normally, but painful or excessive menstruation appears to be more common after laparoscopy.

After sterilization, all that has changed within the body is that when the egg bursts out of the ovary, it cannot reach the end of the Fallopian tube, so it disintegrates and is absorbed by the body. Sexual response is dependent entirely on hormones, the vagina and the clitoris, and is therefore not affected. The operation which does cause permanent sterility, but also cessation of periods and severe menopausal symptoms, is hysterectomy — removal of the womb. (See chapter on this subject.) This should not be confused with the 2 types of sterilization operation we have described here.

## FURTHER READING

*Birth Control Handbook,* (Montreal Health Press)

*Sex with Health; the 'Which' guide to Contraceptives, Abortion and Sex-related diseases,* (Consumers Association 1974)

*Textbook of Contraceptive Practice,* J. Peel and M. Potts, (Cambridge University Press 1969)

*Our Bodies, Ourselves,* ed Angela Phillips and Jill Rakusen, (Penguin 1978)

## ORGANIZATIONS

For your nearest FPA clinic contact:
Family Planning Association, 27-35 Mortimer Street, London W1A 4QW:
Tel 01-636 7866

Brook Advisory Centres are particularly geared for young people. For your nearest branch contact:
Brook Advisory Centres, 233 Tottenham Court Road, London W1P 9AE:
Tel 01-580 2991 and 323 2991

# PREGNANCY TESTING

Quick, easy pregnancy tests were developed in the 1960s. Before that the only tests were 'biological' ones, observing the affect of pregnant blood or urine on the reproduction of animals and usually your GP would tell you to wait until you missed your second period, by which time the signs of pregnancy such as nausea and sore breasts would be apparent in most cases.

But there are many occasions when you need to know as soon as possible so that you can seek ante natal care, avoid drugs or injections that could harm the baby (eg. rubella or smallpox vaccination), get prompt medical care if you have a history of miscarriage or get a safe, early termination.

The pregnancy tests today test for the *human chorionic gonadotropin* (HCG) excreted in your urine. This HCG is produced from the tissue where the egg implants itself in the womb, where the placenta will form. More and more HCG is produced as the pregnancy progresses, reaching a peak between 50 and 90 days after the first day of the last menstrual period and then levelling off. After 3 months the level can vary and it is possible to get 'negative' results at this stage, often around 16 weeks.

The tests in common use can only detect HCG when it reaches a certain concentration; in most women this is when the period is about 2 weeks overdue. At this stage the woman will have been pregnant for a month ie. from the time of ovulation, which is always 2 weeks before the next period, but it will be termed, '6 weeks pregnant', since pregnancy is always dated from the first day of the last menstrual period (LMP), assuming a regular 28-day cycle.

Remember, every woman has an individual level of HCG in pregnancy and some women will show 'positive' on tests before others. You may have to wait until your period is 3 weeks late, or more, so always go back for a re-test if the first result is 'negative'. In the meantime continue to use contraception if you don't want to be pregnant.

60 per cent of women who miss a period and go for a test are not pregnant. It could be Pill amenorrhoea (see chapter on Pill or write to Pam Bingham, 120 Addison Gardens, London W14 0DS for leaflet) stress, illness, travel or the start of the menopause. Keep a chart of your periods, check your ovulation (if you are not on the Pill) remembering that the period always follows ovulation by 2 weeks, because it takes 14 days for the corpus luteum to break down. The 28-day cycle may not apply to you: your cycle is still normal if it is a regular 3, 5 or 6 weeks, or whatever; the length of time *before* ovulation being the variable factor.

If you go to your doctor for a test she/he will probably send a urine sample to the hospital. They will use a 'haemaglutination test' which is done in a test tube and takes a couple of hours. You may have to wait a week for the result because the lab will keep all the samples and do the whole batch at once. Chemists, pregnancy testing agencies and possibly your own GP will use a slide test which takes a few minutes. The tube test is a bit more sensitive and can show positive results a couple of days earlier.

Both the tube and the slide methods are immunological tests and work on the same principle: the woman's urine is added to an antibody to HCG extracted from animals. In the second stage blood cells sensitized with HCG (haemaglutination test) or latex particles coated with HCG (slide test) are added. If the woman has sufficient HCG in her urine, (let's call it 'plus') it will cancel out the anti-HCG ('minus') in stage 1 and nothing further will happen in stage 2. The test is 'positive', indicating pregnancy. This should be confirmed a bit later by pelvic examination. But if there is no, or insufficient, HCG there is no reaction at stage 1, leaving the anti-HCG to react with the HCG particles added at stage 2 and the reaction between them, 'agglutination', indicates a 'negative' result, meaning 'not pregnant' or, 'too early'.

If a test shows 'positive' it is usually right. False results come through human error, out-of-date reagents or washing-up liquid contaminating the sample bottle. (This breaks up the surface tension, preventing agglutination.) If a bench with racks of test tubes is banged the results may become inconclusive. There are many brands of tests and it is possible that some may be affected by drugs in the urine. Gravindex is not so affected and is highly recommended.

Over the last few years it has become possible to detect the extremely low levels of HCG in very early pregnancy, before you've even missed a period, using *radioimmunoassays* (RIAs). They work on the same principle as the other tests but instead of using HCG-coated latex particles or red blood cells the RIAs utilize purified preparations of HCG which have been labelled with radio isotopes of iodine. Reading the results requires skill and expensive equipment.

Beware of the so-called 'hormone withdrawal tests'. Your GP may offer you Primodos or Amenerrone Forte which are high dose progestogen plus oestrogen pills. Repeated doses over a few days will often, but not always, produce bleeding in non-pregnant women when the pills are stopped. This is like withdrawal bleeding on the Pill: it doesn't 'bring on' your period and you may bleed even though you're pregnant. If you are pregnant the hormones may increase the risk of abnormalities in the baby.

It is unwise to rely on home pregnancy testing kits. Not only can they be difficult to read (some depend on distinguishing colour changes and practice in testing definitely leads to less mistakes,) but they may have been stored incorrectly and deteriorated when not refrigerated, or the reagents may be out of date.

The more tests you do the more you realize that there is a whole range of results depending on the amount of HCG present: if a test is done too soon it may be 'inconclusive', it looks neither positive nor negative. As the amount of hormone increases every day the inconclusive test will become a true positive. However, very low or fluctuating levels of HCG may indicate threatened miscarriage or ectopic pregnancy. Very high levels indicate, extremely rarely, cancer or hydatidiform mole (a trophoblastic disease; trophoblastic tissue forms the placenta; the mole is sometimes retained foetal tissue). Pregnancy can only be confirmed by pelvic examination and any unusual test results should be checked at a hospital where they can quantify the amount of HCG.

## ORGANIZATIONS

British Pregnancy Advisory Service: 1st Floor, Guildhall Bldgs, Navigation St, Birmingham 2: Tel Birmingham 643 1461. BPAS has branches in many cities and towns: ask the Birmingham office for your nearest branch.

Release: 1 Elgin Avenue, London W 10: Tel 01-289 1123. Emergency number outside office hours: 01-603 8654.

Brook Advisory Centres: 233 Tottenham Court Rd, London W1P 9AE: Tel 01-580 2991. Again, ask for your nearest branch.

Bristol Women's Centre: 2nd Floor, 59 Union St, Bristol 1: Tel Bristol 22760 Does pregnancy testing and campaigns on aspects of women's health.

Cambridge Pregnancy Advisory Group: 48 Eden St, Cambridge: Tel Cambridge 59798 or 52871 to make an appointment.

Rochdale Women's Group: contact C Bennett, 67 Harewood Rd, Norden, Rochdale, Lans: Tel Rochdale 40878. Free pregnancy tests on Saturdays.

# ABORTION

## REFERRALS

If you have a friendly GP who will refer you to hospital and recommend an abortion, and if you're also lucky enough to get a favourable gynaecologist, you're well on the way to getting a NHS abortion. Although the availability of this operation varies greatly from one region to another, the 1967 Abortion Act has in theory imposed the following standard conditions for the termination of a pregnancy:

Two doctors must agree that

1) continuing the pregnancy involves a greater risk to a woman's life than an abortion; or

2) continuing the pregnancy involves a greater risk of injury to her physical or mental health than an abortion; or

3) continuing the pregnancy involves a greater risk of injury to the physical or mental health of the existing children in the family than an abortion; or

4) there is a substantial risk that the child will be born seriously deformed.

In deciding whether the mental or physical health of the mother or existing children are risked by the pregnancy, doctors may take present or foreseeable future environment into account.

If your attempts are unlucky or you live in one of the many places where it is hard to get an NHS abortion, then you will have to go into the private sector. There are non-profit-making clinics which provide good abortion care together with counselling and contraceptive advice at the lowest prices possible. Commercial clinics will often call themselves by almost the same names, so make sure that you've got the right place.

## METHODS OF ABORTION

### The Morning After Pill

This is a dose of *diethyl stilboestrol* (a hormone) given within 48 hours of 'unprotected' intercourse. It is known to have caused cancer in women who took it in the 1950s, and in their children. (See Menopause chapter.)

### Interception; Termination of Possible Pregnancy; Menstrual Aspiration

This can be done up to 14 days after a period was due. A flexible plastic cannula (tube) only 4-5mm in diameter is passed through the os into the uterus, and the contents sucked out into a syringe attached to the cannula. This is done with a local anaesthetic, but when doctors do it, women tend to find the method very painful. Interception has only been carried out in

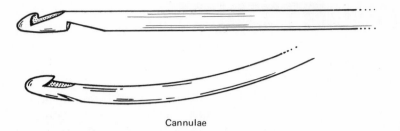

Cannulae

research projects so far, and is not generally available in this country. The advantage of a flexible plastic cannula over a metal curette is that it needs little or no dilatation to pass through the cervix, and is therefore unlikely ) to cause any damage.

### Abortion Under 12 Weeks

This is usually done under general anaesthetic by vacuum aspiration, using a cannula and suction from a machine. When the cannula is used under general anaesthetic, the uterus does not close down round it to indicate that the abortion is complete, so the doctor usually likes to check with a curette. The woman also has to recover from the anaesthetic itself. There are only a very few places doing local anaesthetic abortions on the NHS, and you have to have an address in their catchment area. Pregnancy Advisory Service (PAS) and BPAS have just started doing some 'day care' abortions.

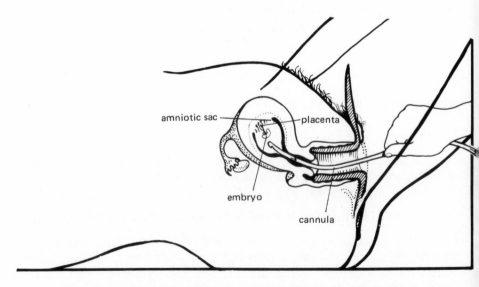

amniotic sac

placenta

embryo

cannula

Vacuum aspiration abortion. This picture shows a different kind of speculum in place

Peter Huntingford, Professor of Obstetrics and Gynaecology and a supporter of a woman's right to choose says that a full abortion service could be provided for women in England and Wales using only 500 part time doctors if day care facilities were made more widely available.

## 12-16 Weeks

A combination of dilatation and curettage and vacuum aspiration is used under general anaesthetic, sometimes with a forceps to help withdraw the foetus. As the matter to be expelled is larger as the days of pregnancy proceed, the cervix has to be dilated to a greater extent, to allow the appropriate instrument to be used. This method carries a higher complication rate. Women *must* have easy access to early abortion.

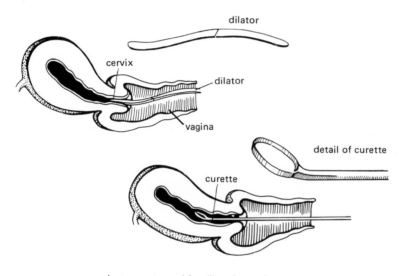

Instruments used for dilatation and curettage

## After 16 Weeks

Abortion can also be induced by setting up a drip containing a hormone (oxytocin) which makes the uterus contract, or by using substances called *prostaglandins,* given by mouth, by intravenous drip into the arm, or by injection into the uterine cavity. There follows a period of 8-15 hours labour, as in childbirth, The knowledge of breathing techniques, to help you relax during the labour pains, may make this period less painful, but you should also have access to pethidine and other pain relief. The foetus is expelled through the cervix and vagina, while the woman is conscious, though she may have been given sedation. This form of abortion may be emotionally difficult, for the procedure of giving birth to a dead foetus, and probably being aware of the hospital staff's distaste for the whole thing, is likely to be very distressing.

## Hysterotomy

With this method the woman is put under a general anaesthetic and the foetus is removed through a small abdominal incision, usually below the pubic hair line. This is major surgery and requires several days' hospitalization and convalescence. A hysterotomy does not affect a woman's reproductive system (unlike *hysterectomy* — the removal of the womb) but it's sometimes necessary to deliver any future child by Caesarean operation, ie. by removing the child through an abdominal incision. Most doctors prefer to avoid hysterotomy for this reason.

## FURTHER READING

*The Lane Report on Abortion*, (HMSO 1974), in 3 vols which you can buy separately — HMSO bookshops.

## CAMPAIGN GROUPS & ORGANIZATIONS

A Woman's Right to Choose (Abortion Law Reform Association): 88a Islington High St, London N18EG: Tel 01-359 5209

National Abortion Campaign: 30 Camden Rd, London NW1:Tel 01-485 4303. Formed to fight restrictive legislation —a co-ordinating committee.

Women's Abortion and Contraception Campaign: c/o Women's Centre, 49 Seel St, Liverpool 1. Contact them for your nearest branch.

# CHILDBIRTH

We do not have a chapter on childbirth, but here is some suggested reading:

*Our Bodies, Ourselves,* ed Angela Phillips and Jill Rakusen, (Penguin 1978)

*The Experience of Childbirth*, Sheila Kitzinger, (Penguin 1970)

*Infant Feeding*, Mavis Gunther, (Penguin 1973)

*Babyhood*, Penelope Leach, (Penguin 1974)

*Birth Without Violence*, Frederick Leboyer, (Wildwood House 1975)

*The Childbirth Book*, Christine Beels (Turnstone 1977)

## ORGANIZATIONS

National Childbirth Trust, 9 Queensborough Terrace, London W2: Tel 01-229 9319
It offers ante natal classes in relaxation and breathing — contact them for your nearest teacher — also has a post natal support system and a breast-feeding promotion group.

Association for Improvements in Maternity Services, Secretary Mrs. A Taylor, West Hill Cottage, Exmouth Place, Hastings, Sussex: Tel Hastings 420591
Produces a newsletter for members; concentrates on improving local facilities.

Society to Support Home Confinements, Margaret Whyte, 17 Laburnam Avenue, Durham City: Tel Durham 61325
Send foolscap s.a.e. for ammunition to fight for home delivery!

London SSHC — for home delivery GPs — Pauline Stephens, 274 Merton Road, London SW 18: Tel 01-874 7940

La Leche League, Secretary Mrs S E McBride, 5 Rose Cottages, Bricket Wood, St Albans, Herts: Tel Garston 74880

# CYSTITIS

Cystitis is the name given to the symptoms of burning pain on passing urine and the urge to go frequently. To cure these symptoms we have first to find the cause or causes — there are many.

If your cystitis attacks start very soon after having intercourse it may be:

## BRUISING

Especially if the woman is a bit dry which often happens with hormonal changes around childbirth, coming on or off the Pill, the menopause and so on. Use KY jelly from the chemist for lubrication.

If your attacks start 12 or 24 hours after having intercourse it's more likely to be:

## INFECTION

Try passing water straight after to flush out any germs that may be there before they get a chance to multiply. One of the commonest bacteria to cause cystitis is called E-coli. This lives in your gut and within moderation that's okay, but not if it gets to your urethra and bladder. To stop it getting there wipe front to back after you have had your bowels open and wash with a flannel and cool water in the same way. Keep the flannel just for that purpose and boil it often. You need to know which kind of bacteria is causing your infection so that you can take the right antibiotic to knock it out. It may take many tests to identify the particular kind. For example some only show up when a culture is grown from the urine and others can only be identified in other ways.

## ALCOHOL

If you want to drink, drink long drinks like beer and drink water too. Herbal tea is good for cystitis sufferers — even if you don't believe in herbs, it's a palatable way of drinking more water.

## WHAT HAPPENS NEXT?

If you have cystitis for a long time, whatever the original cause, the tissues inside your urethra and bladder will become scarred because they have been inflamed for so long. Even if the first cause goes away you may be left with a stricture (blockage) in the system and because it will be difficult to empty the bladder properly you will have a reservoir of urine ready to harbour an infection. Practice stopping and starting the flow when you are peeing — it develops control and means you can still pass water when you have temporarily lost sensation, eg. after childbirth. You may have to have the stricture widened by passing a thin rod up the urethra. If they think the trouble is right inside the bladder they will pass an instrument called a cystoscope to have a look at the bladder walls.

Even if you reach this stage go on with self help and preventive measures to promote the maximum amount of healing possible.

Treat every attack seriously as soon as it starts — drink lots of water and rest so that your body can concentrate on fighting the attack. For more ideas on causes, prevention and first aid for acute bouts of cystitis see the U&I club literature (see below).

## IN MEN

Doctors call it non specific urethritis (non specific meaning they don't know what exactly it is that's inflaming the urethra). Men very often turn up at the VD clinic having picked up the bacteria during sexual intercourse, although the partner may not have any symptoms. It is usually treated with antibiotics and the man is told not to drink alcohol. Sometimes the symptoms subside and if not treated, can develop into pyelonephritis (inflammation of the kidneys, renal pelvis and ureter), which is very painful and if not treated quickly or thoroughly, can permanently damage the kidneys.

## FURTHER READING

*Understanding Cystitis*, Angela Kilmartin (Pan 1975)

## ORGANIZATIONS

U&I Club, 22 Gerrard Road, London N1 8AY: Tel 01-359-0403

# VAGINAL DISCHARGE & VENEREAL DISEASE

## VAGINAL DISCHARGE

This term can be misleading. The discharge comes out of the vagina, but the vagina does not have its own glands. The glands of the cervix put out mucus (clear and watery) which passes down the vagina. Here it picks up dead cells off the vaginal wall and some fluid which oozes from the walls (sometimes very little, other times such as pregnancy, much more). Then it may be joined by the juice produced by the glands at the entrance to the vagina when a woman gets sexually excited.

A lot of women have some discharge all the time or during one particular part of their monthly cycle. This is normal. When a discharge causes irritation — itchiness and soreness and/or has an unpleasant smell, there is probably something wrong.

## WHAT COULD IT BE?

### Don't Forget Foreign Bodies

A lot of women forget to remove things they put into their vaginas — usually tampax (or other internal tampons). This can cause a really thick, bad smelly discharge. It will clear up as soon as the object is completely removed and after a good wash.

### Deodorants and Disinfectants

Vaginal deodorants usually in spray form cause a lot of women soreness and discharge. The sensitive skin is reacting to the very strong chemicals in the spray. Using disinfectants (like Dettol) in your bathwater can make you sore. Don't be too harsh on yourself.

### After the Menopause

Many years after periods have stopped women may suffer from vaginal discharge, irritation or soreness. This may be due to a low level of oestrogen in the body. Doctors often prescribe oestrogen pills and the discharge clears up. Oestrogen is produced by the ovaries in women still ovulating and having periods. It is oestrogen that normally keeps the vagina acid. So maybe you could try a simple cure to try to make the vagina more acid. (See under Thrush.)

# Infection

Infections that most commonly cause vaginal discharge are Thrush, Trichomonas vaginalis, and gonorrhoea (for Trichomonas and gonorrhoea see under VD).

## THRUSH

Thrush (otherwise known as monilia, candida albicans, or yeast infection) is very common and is caused by a type of fungus, a yeast. The yeast is normally found in the vagina but the normal acid conditions in the vagina do not encourage its growth. At certain times, conditions in the vagina change and the yeast thrives and multiplies. This causes a thick, creamy discharge which can make a woman very itchy and sore, inside and outside. The discharge may smell 'yeasty' and inside the vagina you can see white patches sticking to the walls, looking like cottage cheese. You are more likely to get Thrush if you are pregnant, taking the contraceptive Pill, taking antibiotics (such as penicillin) or have sugar diabetes. All these tend to make the vaginal walls more sugary and less acid, so the yeast can grow.

Thrush is not normally caught from anyone else (through sex) but it can be, so if you get it again and again, it might be from your partner. Men normally have no symptoms, but may get a discharge and/or pain with pissing – Thrush may be growing under the foreskin. Repeated infections of Thrush may be the first sign that you have developed sugar diabetes – this is a serious disease, but one that can be controlled well with contant supervision. Go and get a check up.

*Prevention*
To help prevent Thrush keep vaginal area dry and airy, wear cotton pants (or none under a skirt), avoid nylon tights, tight trousers; wash with plain water or soap without deodorant or perfume; and wipe your bottom from front to back.

*Treatment*
Standard treatment from the doctor is with Nystatin (Nystan) pessaries (big tablets you push right up to the top of the vagina). The usual dose is 1 a night for 1 week or 2, and it is usually very effective. (Don't use tampons with pessaries, as they absorb all the Nystatin and stop it touching the thrush; but wear an old pair of pants or a pad, because it will stain things yellow.) You can   stop Thrush by making the vagina more acid again. Some women use yogurt. Any natural yogurt will do – put it in tampax inserters, contraceptive foam inserter with plunger or put in a speculum and apply the yogurt with a spoon. If you catch the Thrush early, you need only use it once or twice. I soaked myself in a bowl of warm water with 2 or 3 tablespoons of vinegar in it. After 3 days of 2 soaks a day, the Thrush cleared up.

Some women use herbs (1 oz dried herb to 1 pint water, simmer 10 mins, cool) soaking in bowl or using a douche, eg. Goldenseal, Calendula (Marigold), sage, thuja.

## VENEREAL DISEASE, VD, OR SEXUALLY TRANSMITTED DISEASES

VD means different things to different people. Venereal diseases are spread from one person to another during sexual intercourse. There are many different diseases; they are all contagious and each disease is caused by a germ, which usually enters your body during sexual intercourse. Some venereal diseases are serious, others are not; but most can be cured if diagnosed early. Many of the diseases don't produce any symptoms. In other words, you don't know you've got them, so *it is important* if you know you have a sexually transmitted disease (VD) to tell your sex partners. The chances are high that they will have it too and not know about it. It is also important to remember you may have more than one disease. When you identify one and treat it, another may pass undetected and you may end up with complications. For example, you may have Trichomonas and gonorrhoea and suffer a vaginal discharge, itchiness and soreness. You go to your own doctor: he does no tests but gives you a prescription for 'Flagyl Compac'. This is a combination pack of tablets taken by mouth, to cure Trichomonas, and vaginal tablets to cure Thrush. This means that if you have either Trichomonas or Thrush, or both, the discharge and irritation will go. The danger is if you have Trichomonas and gonorrhoea: this treatment will clear up the Trichomonas and all the symptoms – but you will be left with the gonorrhoea; and in one third of women, gonorrhoea produces no discharge or discomfort at all, at first. Then later on (maybe a few months later), you may end up in hospital very ill and perhaps sterile. This is one advantage of special VD clinics. They do a thorough examination and a whole range of tests to cover all kinds of sexually transmitted diseases. They usually do follow-up tests within a week or 2 of the first visit to check if any disease that has been treated is cured and to make sure any other diseases have not gone undiscovered. GPs don't know much about VD and may do tests that will dectect one disease but not another. (Legally, only 3 diseases are called venereal diseases – syphilis, gonorrhoea and chancroid – only common in the tropics – so you may have a disease spread by sexual intercourse but be told that you haven't got VD.) Here are some of the most common diseases.

## TRICHOMONAS VAGINALIS

This is caused by a one-celled microscopic animal called Trichomonas vaginalis (TV or Trich). It is the commonest cause of vaginal discharge. 50 per cent of women with gonorrhoea also have TV. 45 per cent of women who have tests for a discharge when they are pregnant turn out to have TV. The discharge is yellow with pus; it smells unpleasant and makes the inside and outside of the vagina very sore. The discharge comes from the os of the cervix and looks frothy. Raised red spots in clusters are often seen on the cervix and vaginal walls (raspberry effect).

*Treatment*

TV tends to thrive in a less acid vagina, like Thrush, so simple treatment to make the vagina more acid can be tried (see treatment of Thrush). The doctor will prescribe Flagyl (Metronidazole) tablets – either a 7 day course of 2 tablets (200mg) 3 times a day or a single dose of 2G. These are usually very effective; do not take Flagyl if you are pregnant or breastfeeding. (Food & Drug Research Council in USA are reviewing Flagyl – it is found to lower the body's resistance to infection by a temporary decrease in the number of white cells in the blood.)

Don't drink alcohol while taking Flagyl as you may be very sick. Flagyl is very strong and can effect the acid balance of your vagina giving you Thrush. Sometimes Flagyl or Penotrane pessaries are used but these may not be so effective. Women's health groups are using a clove of garlic put into the vagina and left overnight.

Adelle Davis suggests 6mg Vitamin B2 and Vitamin B6 per day (and Vitamin B6 salve). Herbs some women use include Motherwort as a drink (1 teaspoon/cup water) will relieve itching, Pure Alum for a soak or a douche (1 teaspoon/pint water), Inner bark of Oak, to soak or douche (1oz bark/pint water), Slippery Elm to drink or douche (2 teaspoons/cup – not when you're pregnant), Stinging Nettle Tea or douche (4 tablespoons/cup boiled for 20 mins).

These may help with itching and soreness, but not clear up TV properly; worth trying (especially Vitamin B6) if you are pregnant or can't take Flagyl, or have done but without success.

*Spread*

TV is usually passed on by intercourse. Men may get pain on pissing, or maybe a discharge, but more often they don't suffer at all. So if the woman gets TV again and again when sleeping with the same man then he should get treatment too.

Remember that half the women who have gonorrhoea also have TV. Having the symptoms of TV cleared up does not necessarily mean that you are also free of the gonorrhoea. If you go for a check up don't wash out your vagina before you go, as this may obscure the symptoms.

## GONORRHOEA

This is caused by bacteria called *gonococci*. Women sometimes get a vaginal discharge, pain on pissing and pissing more frequently. Men nearly always get a very obvious discharge from the penis and burning when pissing. The incubation period is usually 3 to 10 days, but may be as long as 3 weeks. In other words the symptoms develop (you get the discharge) 3 to 10 days after contact. But one third of women with gonorrhoea have no symptoms at all. Half the women with gonorrhoea also have TV (see above) and it is usually TV which gives you the discharge. The TV may be cured while the gonorrhoea remains undetected. This means that you pass on the disease to your sex partners and that serious complications can develop meanwhile.

*Complications*
The infection can spread from the cervix through the uterus or womb into the Fallopian tubes. The tubes get infected and inflamed and you get severe pain, feel feverish and often feel sick. These symptoms are often mistaken for acute appendicitis and not discovered until a healthy appendix has been removed by emergency operation. Like appendicitis if not dealt with, the disease can lead to peritonitis and may be fatal. Inflammation of the tubes (known as salpingitis) leaves a scar which may cause a blockage or a narrowing of the Fallopian tubes. If both sides of the tubes are blocked, no sperm can get to the eggs to fertilize them so the woman is sterile. If the tube or tubes are narrowed the egg may be fertilized but can't get down to the tube to the womb. This can mean a pregnancy developing outside the womb (an ectopic pregnancy) and this can be very dangerous.

*Treatment*
The simplest and most effective treatment is with penicillin. The dose varies from place to place. Within Britain the doses will vary only a little, usually depending which doctor prescribes it. But in different countries, eg. USA,Vietnam, the dose will have to be much higher because the strain of bacteria has become very resistant to the penicillin. The penicillin is usually given by injection into the muscle of your bottom or leg (eg. 1.2-2.4 megaunits Procaine Penicillin). Penicillin works very fast and effectively when given by injection. For people allergic or sensitive to penicillin, the most effective alternative antibiotics are Kanamycin or Erythromycin. If you are taking a week's course of penicillin tablets (or must go back to the doctor for a second injection) it is advisable to finish the whole course of tablets (or go for that injection). Taking half a course means the bacteria which are strongest don't get destroyed, they spread and get stronger and a new strain grows up which is more resistant to the penicillin, which needs huge doses of penicillin to destroy it.

*Tests*
When you go for tests, don't wash your vagina or have a soak just before you go because they might not find it even if it is there. Swabs should be taken from the cervical os (hole in the cervix) and from the urinary open-

ing (the opening from your bladder where the urine comes from), so you should not pass urine just before the test. A swab taken just from high up in the vagina (a high vaginal swab or HVS) will not pick up the gonorrhoea.

## SYPHILIS

Syphilis is caused by bacteria called Treponema Pallidum (or Spirochete). The incidence of syphilis is declining but it is a serious disease, with long term results including paralysis, 'madness', and heart disease. It is very rare for syphilis to be passed on any way other than during sexual intercourse.

### Signs and Symptoms of Syphilis

There are four stages of this disease:

*Primary (or first) Stage*
This stage may show itself after 1 week, or not until 3 months after having intercourse with an infected person. (This is why VD clinics ask you to go back for follow up tests.) Usually about 3 or 4 weeks after getting infected a primary sore or chancre appears at the spot where the bacteria have got into your body. In women, it is normally on the cervix, vaginal walls or the vaginal lips; in men on the penis or scrotum (balls). It can appear on the lips, tongue or throat after oral intercourse (sucking your lover's penis or vagina). *The sore is painless* so in women it usually goes unnoticed. Men often see the sore but it is painless for them too. If left untreated the sore heals within 1 to 6 weeks but the person is still infectious.

*Secondary Stage*
About 6 weeks (it can range from 2 weeks to 6 months) after the primary sore first appears, a rash all over the body starts. *This rash does not itch or hurt.* In the warm, damp parts of the body, such as the vaginal lips and the anus (back passage), some people get growths like large, flat, warts called 'condylomata lata'. Usually the rash or 'warts' are obvious and will mean that you will get treatment from the doctor and you will recover completely. But even with no treatment the rash (and warts) will go away after a few weeks. You may then think you have recovered but the untreated syphilis then gets to the third, hidden stage.

*Latent (hidden) Stage*
This stage has no symptoms and may last many years (20 to 30 years). After about 1 year in this stage the disease is no longer infectious. About two thirds of people who never get treatment don't suffer any more, but one third go on to the late stage of syphilis.

*Late Syphilis*
There are 3 kinds of late syphilis; benign, cardiovascular and neurosyphilis.
1) Benign late syphilis: About 5 years after catching the syphilis, a des-

tructive ulcer can form and gradually eat away the skin, eyes, lungs or many other parts of the body. If you are treated at this stage, you can recover and the disease will stop.

2) Cardiovasular syphilis: This affects the heart and major blood vessels from 10 to 40 years after catching syphilis. It is often the cause of death.

3) Neurosyphilis: This affects the spinal cord and/or the brain. It can cause paralysis, but usually means the person ends up very slow and incapable of looking after herself/himself (called general paralysis of the insane, GPI). Treatment can stop the disease going any further but complete recovery is rare. Late syphilis is very rare in Britain nowadays.

### Finding Syphilis — Tests

Detecting or diagnosing syphilis is difficult. Signs and symptoms are so often missed or mistaken for another disease. If there is a sore, rash or wart, then a bit is scraped off and looked at under a microscope. The bacteria can be seen and identified. But if none of these are present, a blood test must be done. Blood is taken from a vein and several tests done. The blood test doesn't pick up syphilis until after 6 weeks, so it must be repeated to be reliable. The disease may not show itself for 3 months after the germs get into the person's body, so the blood tests might not be positive until 4 months after sleeping with the 'infected' person.

### Treatment of Syphilis

Treatment by injection of penicillin into the muscle (leg or bottom). The amount varies with each stage. The course of penicillin should be completed and follow up test should also be done to make sure the disease is cured.

### In Pregnancy

Syphilis can be passed on by a pregnant woman to her unborn child. Generally the more recent the infection the more likely it is that the baby will get infected. It is Treponema Pallidum (the germ or bacteria) in the woman's blood that passes through to the baby's blood. In the first 4 months of pregnancy the baby is not affected, so preferably treatment of the syphilis in a pregnant woman should be in the first 4 months. If the woman is not infected, or not treated until later on in pregnancy, the baby should be cured and will be born healthy.

## MISCELLANEOUS INFECTIONS—WARTS (GENITAL/VENEREAL)

These are caused by a virus similar to the virus which causes warts on the fingers and feet. They are often passed on through sexual intercourse, but *not* always. Since they thrive in a similar environment to Thrush, they tend to come in pregnancy *and* when taking the Pill. Jenny had warts that kept on coming back even after surgery, and as soon as she stopped the Pill they went and have never returned. So change the environment — it might work (see Thrush). Warts can be on the cervix, in the vagina, outside the lips and around the anus (back passage). They are usually itchy.

*Treatment*
1) By painting Podophyllum in spirit on the warts twice a week. You have to get this from the doctor. You can buy ointment called Pasatfilin at the chemist. This must be done with care because the normal skin around the warts may be very sensitive to the Podophyllum — if it gets sore stop the treatment. Some warts respond well, some don't. If your warts don't respond, insist on some alternative treatment.

2) Warts on the outside of the vaginal lips can be removed by freezing the skin locally (with ethyl chloride spray) and scraping them off with a Volkmann's spoon.

3) Warts inside the vagina, or on the cervix or a bit too big to be scraped off should be removed by diathermy (they are burnt off with a needle) under an anaesthetic. Some warts are connected with secondary syphilis (see above).

4) Recurrent warts — either find out who they are coming from *or* change that environment (see Thrush).

## HERPES GENITALIS

This is caused by a virus Herpes 2 (Herpes 1 causes cold sores) and is found on the cervix, in the vagina and on the inner and outer vaginal lips. It starts with itching, then little blisters appear which break and become very sore.

Attacks of herpes tend to recur, but the first attack is always the most painful. There is no cure, but various ways are tried to relieve the soreness. Keeping still helps, so stay in bed; cold used tea bags applied to the sore, or try lignocaine ointment, bathing several times a day with a cupful of salt in the bath (this guards against secondary infection too). Herpes can make you feel very ill all over. Painkillers such as paracetamol and aspirin may relieve the pain. (A sore is a sign of syphilis so you might need tests to make sure you haven't got syphilis.)

In a pregnant woman an active herpes infection (ie.presence of a sore) can seriously affect the baby *at delivery*, so a Caesarian section may be needed. Recently Herpes 2 virus has been thought to be connected with cervical cancer. This does not mean that most women with genital herpes get cervical cancer, but it is important to have a smear once a year.

The virus is found in men who have no symptoms, and so herpes is often passed on during sexual intercourse.

## CRABS (PEDICULOSIS PUBLIS — PUBIC LICE)

Pubic lice infest the pubic hair (sometimes the hair under the armpits and
the eyebrows) and cause severe itching.
They are usually passed on through
intercourse. The lice lay the eggs at the
root of the hairs, these are the nits and
are difficult to remove.

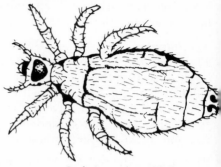

Body Louse (magnified)

*Treatment*
Treatment is with DDT (Dicophane)
emulsion or powder. The hair is best
not shaved off. If the hair is left it will absorb a little of the DDT and kill off
the nits. Other powders are sometimes used. The emulsion can cause a bad
skin reaction in some people. Try just a little first before coating yourself.

## SCABIES

This is a very infectious disease passed on by any intimate contact (such as
holding hands). It causes an itchy rash between the fingers, on the wrists
and around the genitals (and many other places).

*Treatment*
Treatment is with Benzyl Benzoate emulsion. All bedding, towels and
clothes must be changed and cleaned. All the people in the house or house-
hold should be treated.

## MOLLUSCUM CONTAGIOSUM

This is caused by a virus and results in little wartlike bumps the size of a
large pinhead with a dip in the centre. It usually occurs on the genitals,
face and shoulders. The incubation period can be up to 6 months, and they
are treated by putting phenol on the centre of the bump.

## FURTHER READING

*VD Handbook*, (Montreal Health Press)

Medical textbooks on VD

VD leaflets — available from Family Planning Association and Health
Education Council

*The Monthly Extract*, Box 3488, Ridgeway Station, Stamford, Connecti-
cut 06905, USA (especially good on herpes — vol 4 issue 3 Oct/Nov 1975;
vol 5 issue 2 July/Aug 1976

# HYSTERECTOMY

'In a woman who has had her family, the uterus is a foreign body and should be removed,' American gynaecologist quoted in the *American Journal of Obstetrics and Gynaecology.*

'Women who have had hysterectomies are 4 times more likely to become depressed within three years than women who have not,' British GP in the *Lancet.*

Hysterectomy — an operation to remove the uterus — is the second commonest operation in women. Many women who have had cancer owe their lives, perhaps unknowingly, to a hysterectomy. Many more, relieved of heavy bleeding and great discomfort, are grateful for the operation, take on a new lease of life, and say they have 'never felt better'.

## HYSTERECTOMY AS PROFIT MAKING

The first thing that struck me when I started reading some of the innumerable articles in medical journals, particularly American ones, was the uncanny *enthusiasm* with which some gynaecologists discussed the subject. It is an attitude not entirely accounted for by the profits of private health care, although many an American doctor must have bought a Cadillac on the proceeds of womb disposal. Nearly thirty years ago Dr Norman Miller embarrassed fellow medics in an article titled 'Hysterectomy — therapeutic procedure or surgical racket?' in which he wrote of the 'chronic remunerative or hip-pocket hysterectomy'. Only last year a Senator commented: 'If you've got Blue Cross insurance, they'll have your uterus.' A recent article by a Professor of Social Medicine pointed out that it was impossible to assess the effectiveness of screening for cancer of the cervix because such a high percentage of North American females no longer had one.

## ABORTION & STERILIZATION

But it is not just the rich and insured who may have an unnecessary operation. Some American doctors are becoming enthusiastic advocates of vaginal hysterectomy as 'the ideal abortion for the indigent multiparous patient' (in other words poor women with lots of kids who get free medical care). Some of them are as young as 21. Doctors say these women are unlikely to come back for check-ups, and will therefore be saved from the possibility of future disease. But they are also unlikely to get oestrogen replacement therapy if they develop severe menopausal symptoms which will make it harder to cope with poverty and kids.

Perhaps we should send our American sisters copies of the Lane Committee Report on the Working of the Abortion Act (£4.74 for 3 fascinating volumes from HMSO) which found that a hysterectomy is the most dangerous kind of abortion you can have and should never be performed without good reason. 'Hysterectomy performed at a gestation of less than 13 weeks carried a death rate up to 5 times higher than that of any other group: this is particularly striking in the over 30 year old age group.'

The Lane Committee warning is timely. Only 5 of 32 patients who had a termination hysterectomy in a British hospital had uterine disease. It was suggested that if the women had been sterilized merely by tying Fallopian tubes, they might have needed a hysterectomy later, because 17 per cent of women who had had a tubal ligation needed a hysterectomy within the next 10 years! But this means that 83 per cent did not — a poor argument (and an expensive one for the NHS) for removing everyone's uterus.

## AFTER EFFECTS & SEXUALITY

The effects of hysterectomy on a woman's sex life are seldom mentioned, let alone dealt with from her point of view. Far too little honest information is given to patients on possible effects on libido — which can increase with fear of unwanted pregnancy removed, remain unchanged, or disappear disastrously during a premature menopause. Women also want to know about the sheer physical aspects — size and shape of the vagina (a number of women in one area claimed theirs was now too short), lubrication, effect of removal of the cervix. Although a subtotal hysterectomy (leaving the cervix) can be done, a total hysterectomy is most commonly carried out. Few women know this, or have exchanged information on comparative effects. Doctors fear that if the cervix remains and cancer develops later it will be difficult to deal with. The more medical literature you read, the more you realize that the priorities of any individual woman may be very different from those of her male doctors. 'Occasionally a patient complains that the loss of the cervix has effected her libido during coitus but an assurance

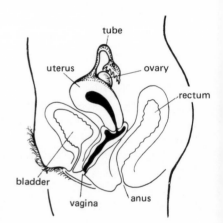

Before a hysterectomy

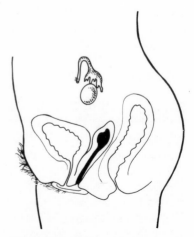

After a hysterectomy. In this case the tubes and ovaries have been left behind.

82

that a possible cancer bearing area has been removed should be enough to
satisfy her ...' (come to think of it, male genitalia are also potentially
cancer bearing areas!)

## AFTER EFFECTS & EMOTIONAL ATTITUDES

The fact that psychiatric illness is more common in women who have had
hysterectomies than amongst the female population as a whole is common
knowledge in the medical profession. But this is usually attributed to the
fact that these women were more 'neurotic' in the first place. A whole list
of female ailments have, for example, been attributed to pre-existing
neuroses in the women concerned. It is suggested that any problems
resulting from hysterectomy could 'be analyzed and controlled by the
stable and intelligent woman'.

Some consultants say that 'patients with gynaecological complaints are
particularly prone to be psychologically unstable' and that their illness is
often 'a psychic conflict sailing under a gynaecological flag'. In this case,
surely the NHS should be providing cheaper, and more effective health
care by referring such patients to a sympathetic female psychotherapist
rather than adding them to lengthy waiting lists and giving them an expensive and apparently unnecessary operation when resources are stretched to
the limit?

## ASKING FOR HYSTERECTOMIES

Doctors claim that some women beg for unnecessary hysterectomies, and
that others who need an operation are reluctant because the uterus has
'unnecessary significance to the patient for her own self image of woman-
liness'. Doubtless both kinds of patient exist, but the answer is not as
some of them imply — that all would be well if only women were more
docile in accepting medical advice, but that women must educate themselves to understand the choices and problems in their own terms.

It is, I suspect, the gynaecologists — male and female — who actually like
women as people, who are most successful in achieving mutual communication with their patients.

However desperately a woman needs a hysterectomy, a doctor may refuse to operate if her husband does not give written permission, and some
nurses have told me of their deep embarrassment at having to get such forms
signed. One told me last year that a severely ill patient was sent home because her husband refused to sign — on the grounds that he wanted more
children.

# RESEARCH IN RECENT YEARS

18 years ago a woman doctor Katharine Dalton (author of *The Menstrual Cycle*) presented a paper at the Royal Society of Medicine suggesting how seriously the emotional complications of hysterectomy might be in some women. She did not claim that her practice was typical, since women with 'female complaints' were over-represented, but she had found that 44 per cent had marital problems after hysterectomies. 'Undoubtedly in many cases marital discord may have been present before hysterectomy, but this vital event in the lives of a married couple may possibly prove to be the last straw'.

She was probably the first researcher to suggest that the percentage of women dissatisfied with the operation *increased* over time (later substantiated by other researchers) so that gynaecologists who congratulated themselves on the high percentage of satisfied patients at post-operation check up (as many still do) had underestimated the after effects. Less than 1 year after the operation 83 per cent were satisfied, but this fell to 41 per cent between 1 and 5 years afterwards. Those who had ovaries removed were more likely to be dissatisfied than those who had not. Patients complained of vertigo, hot flushes, rheumatism, lethargy, depression and weight gain. She suggested that for some patients alternative forms of treatment should be considered first.

14 years later a major British study on psychiatric illness after hysterectomy by Dr Montagu Barker was published. It was based on over 700 women who were compared with a control group who had had another operation. The hysterectomy group were more likely to be referred to a psychiatrist (7 per cent against 3 per cent) and referral *for the first time* was 5 times as common (5 per cent and 1 per cent). The peak time for referral was 2 years after the operation. Women who had had a previous psychiatric illness were more than 10 times as likely to have a further illness after hysterectomy.

Barker did not find a higher referral rate among those who also had ovaries removed. Women with organic disease (cancer, fibroids or ovarian tumours) were *less* likely to have psychiatric problems than those who had not. But those without serious physical cause for hysterectomy were also more likely to have had previous psychiatric treatment, and were therefore more vulnerable. This relationship between absence of serious physical disease and higher risk of mental illness has been noted in other studies.

The Barker study did not include psychiatric illness treated by GPs, and it was a general practitioner – Dr D H Richards – who provided the next, and possibly very significant, link in a study published in 1974. Of 200 women who had had a hysterectomy, he found that 36.5 per cent had been treated by their doctors for depression. Older women were less at risk, but in women under 40 it rose to 55 per cent. Although hysterectomy patients were more likely to have had depression before the operation than the control group, even if those previously treated were excluded, the comparative rates were 24 per cent and 5 per cent. Moreover depression in the hysterectomy group lasted longer — around 2 years compared with 11 months for the controls. He, too, found that patients with more serious conditions were *less* likely to have depression. Those most likely to become depressed were those who had suffered from dysfunctional bleeding. In more than half the women who became depressed, no abnormality was found at the operation.

Richards concluded: The effect of hysterectomy seems in some respects to resemble that of the menopause but in an exaggerated form.

He pointed out that many women start having hot flushes even though the ovaries remain, and suggested that 'This and other symptoms raise the possibility that an endocrine factor may be involved even when the uterus alone is removed.' This is a potentially revolutionary suggestion since the generally held view is that there is no clear evidence that the uterus has a general metabolic or endocrine function — in other words its removal does not fundamentally affect a women's body chemistry.

Many — perhaps most — gynaecologists will strongly disagree with Richards' interpretation. But one thing is indisputable: as the number of hysterectomies performed each year increases, so will mental illness among the female population. The number of 'potentially cancer bearing' organs will be reduced, but some women — and their families — will be paying a price. The price may not be depression alone. Hysterectomy has been linked with both a higher crime rate and a higher accident rate. When Dr Dalton studied women admitted to a London hospital after accidents, she found an unduly high proportion who had had a hysterectomy and suggested that 'Women who have had an artificial menopause appear more accident prone than those whose menopause was natural'. Professor Gibbens of the Institute of Psychiatry in a study of female crime reported that the typical shoplifter 'is a woman of 50 who a year before had a hysterectomy and has not felt well since. She has backaches, headaches, dizziness, insomnia and a persistent sense of depression'.

It seems to be increasingly common to remove the ovaries when taking out the uterus (referred to in medical journals as 'castration' in case you didn't know!) even if there is no sign of disease, particularly if the woman is nearing menopausal age. This again is to 'prevent further trouble' for if cancer subsequently develops it will be hard to detect. A woman who had a hysterectomy recently told me she was the only patient in the ward who kept her ovaries — but only because she asked beforehand if it was to be done and refused to allow it. Many gynaecologists, however, oppose unnecessary 'oophorectomy' and ask if it is right to remove the ovaries of a 100 women to prevent cancer developing in 1. In up to 50 per cent of women the ovaries continue to produce oestrogen long after the menopause, and this helps to protect them both from cardiovascular disease and brittle bones. If ovaries have to be removed, an oestrogen implant can be inserted at the time of the operation to prevent menopausal symptoms; without this 85 per cent of women develop severe hot flushes. But it would seem sensible to preserve as much ovarian tissue as possible and not unnecessarily substitute an artificial implant for a woman's natural hormones. Richards found that women with hormone implants were no less likely to get depression.

The lessons would seem to be:

1) Any unusual bleeding *must be investigated* .

2) Make sure your hysterectomy is really necessary, particularly if you are reasonably young, have ever needed psychiatric treatment, and doctors can find no evidence of organic disease.

There is clear evidence of a relationship between heavy blood loss not caused by obvious disease, marital stress and mental illness before and after hysterectomy. Exactly how these are interrelated we do not know and it is a question to which gynaecologists do not have the answer and which women themselves should explore.

Meantime, the makers of Valium and Librium are doing very nicely ...

# CANCER IN WOMEN

A woman has a 5 per cent chance of getting cancer of the breast.
A woman has a 2 per cent chance of getting cancer of the cervix.
A woman has a 1 per cent chance of getting cancer of the womb.

The word cancer means 'crab'. Probably the name was chosen because a cancer seems to reach out like the claws of a crab, and spread through the body. A cancer consists of a group of cells which differ from the ordinary cells in the body in that, instead of growing in an orderly, controlled way to become healthy tissue, they seem to be out of control and spread rapidly through the body, either in the blood or straight through the tissue, killing the normal cells as they grow. Because they grow so fast, they often run out of food and energy, and some may die, causing ulcers (NB most ulcers – stomach ulcers for instance – are not cancerous. Cancer ulcers are usually buried somewhere in the body and only show themselves as a general feeling of illness and weakness). Because the cancerous cells use a lot of food, people with cancer often lose weight.

As advanced cancer is so difficult to deal with, most research now is directed towards prevention and early treatment: for instance, the discouragement of smoking as a preventive measure against lung cancer.

In some cases, cancer has been known simply to disappear of its own accord. It is said that people can cure themselves by willpower: this may be rare, but is surely possible. The main thing is not to despair, and above all, not to be too frightened to seek treatment or advice if you are worried.

## CANCER OF THE BREAST

We are treating this in most detail because it is the most common cancer in women.

### Is Early Detection Important?

A London surgeon expresses one extreme: 'If breast cancer is caught reasonably early, the woman has about an 80 per cent chance of survival and enjoying a normal life span. If she is caught very early, and the lump is a fairly simple one, her chances are about 95 per cent.' The Women's National Cancer Control Campaign (WNCCC) takes a similar view on the treatment of 'early' cases, citing an 80 per cent success rate (by 'early' they mean before the lymph nodes under the arm are affected or heavily affected).

At the other extreme we find Ivan Illich, author of *Medical Nemesis*, an extensive, much publicized critique of the medical profession. He attempts to show that there is no difference in survival rates between treated and untreated breast cancer.

## Symptoms of Breast Cancer

Symptoms of breast cancer are: a painless lump in the breast – usually in the upper, outer part; swelling of one breast which persists after or between periods; dimpling of the skin of the breast – a sort of puckered appearance; gradual inversion or pulling in of one nipple in someone who has not had this before (some people have inverted nipples naturally); bleeding from the nipple – not during breast feeding; soreness of one nipple with flaking of the skin lasting more than 1 month.

## How is Early Detection Possible?

1) Regular self-examination: women are better than ordinary doctors at finding lumps in their own breasts. If a woman makes an effort to get to know her breasts, and examines them regularly, she is in an ideal position to distinguish any changes. (See chapter on Breast Self Examination.)

2) Clinical examination: detailed and skilled manual examination by trained personnel.

3) At present there are 2 other screening techniques which form important back-ups to manual examination. These are *thermography* (infra red thermographic examination) and *mammography* (X ray). Thermography is a safe and painless technique which involves cooling the skin and with the help of a machine, examining the contours of the breast. Mammography involves a small X-ray exposure. Neither technique is perfect. Thermography can produce a considerable number of false positive results and for this reason has been found unsuitable for use on the general population. In fact, many people now think that it is virtually useless. While mammography is particularly useful in detecting lumps in women past the menopause, for other women it cannot apparently do much better than detecting tumours which a skilled manual examination should be able to catch.

However, as both thermography and mammography can detect lumps before they can be felt (at this stage there is the greatest chance of curing the disease), all 3 techniques of clinical examination are useful. Mammography and skilled manual examination and possibly thermography should be available to women at risk, eg. women over 50, those with a history of breast cancer on their mother's side or women who have had non-malignant breast disease. Mammography should not be used on all women because of the danger from the X ray itself. For this reason, it is now thought that contrary to previous opinion, women between 40 and 50 who are otherwise not at risk (apart from their age) should not be subjected to regular mammographic screening.

Diagnosis of breast cancer cannot be made by your average or even better than average clinic doctor or GP. It can only be confirmed by a biopsy report and women should insist on this as soon as possible – or other women should insist on their sisters' behalf.

# Treatment

So far, the possibilities in orthodox medicine are as follows:

1) removal of the lump alone (*lumpectomy*)

2) removal of the breast alone (*simple mastectomy*)

3) removal of the breast and some lymph nodes under the arm (*modified radical mastectomy*)

4) removal of the breast, chest wall muscles beneath it — which is much more deforming than the above — and the lymph nodes (*radical*)

Together with each of the above operations, drug therapy or radiotherapy may be given.

5 years ago, 90 per cent of women were given radicals, in spite of evidence published in the 1960s that they were not necessarily more effective and were in some cases less so. I have talked to several people about the situation in Britain. The director of the Cancer Intelligence unit for the West of Scotland thinks that most surgeons are tending towards 'conservative' surgery (ie. conserving as much as possible), and this is borne out by the experience of Betty Westgate of the Mastectomy Association. Graham Bennette of the British Cancer Council could not think of anyone who would recommend a 'Halsted' radical nowadays; the more deforming and disabling radical operations, as done in the USA, are scarcely ever done here. Radical operations were recently performed on Betty Ford and Happy Rockefeller: they emerged from their operations smiling, waving their arms above their heads, and this in no small way accounts for the fact that breast clinics in Britain as well as the USA became inundated with women coming forward for tests and treatment.

While radical operations of some description are still performed, simple mastectomies are the most usual operations in Britain. Work is going on with even smaller operations, but there are very real pros and cons attached to lumpectomies. In a small proportion of women, the breast can be saved either by performing a lumpectomy or simply using radiotherapy; the stage, kind and place of the tumour are all crucial (lumpectomies are more feasible if the tumour is not in the outer part of the breast, and of course only feasible if diagnosis is made early). One difficulty at present is deciding when lumpectomy or simple radiotherapy alone is possible; it is much easier to tell when they are not possible.

Difficulties are compounded by the problems attached to accurate diagnosis. For instance, there is some degree of difficulty attached to diagnosing whether or not the cancer has spread to the lymph nodes; such knowledge is crucial if 'conservative' treatment is envisaged. One can also find that different parts of a tumour are in different stages of development. Furthermore, not all pathologists agree on whether certain cell conditions are cancer or not. It seems that in the USA they are more liberal with the term; in fact, one has to continually bear in mind that 'cancer' in one country might not be the same disease as 'cancer' in another country. Obviously, a lumpectomy can only be considered if there is no doubt about diagnosis and all other relevant factors.

## Diagnosis

You've probably guessed that diagnosis difficulties can lead to mistakes: pathologists could diagnose as cancer borderline cases or cases where they were uncertain, in order to protect themselves from giving a false negative diagnosis. Unnecessary mastectomies do occur, particularly with difficult diagnosis, although it is obviously difficult to establish exactly how common such mistakes are. The risk of such mistakes occurring can of course be minimized. For example, in some places it is standard practice for a 'frozen' biopsy to be done, taken to the laboratory and diagnosed while the woman is still under the anaesthetic, and further surgery is then carried out if the decision is 'positive'. In this situation, the pathologist is under pressure to make a quick decision while the woman remains unconscious. If there is no such pressure, the pathologist can make a less hasty decision with the possibility of doing more tests, and surgery can then be carried out a few days later, if need be. The wait of a few days makes absolutely no difference in terms of safety, although it is more demanding on NHS resources in terms of time and staff.

You might have heard of office biopsies which do not require a general anaesthetic. Ellen Frankfort (author of *Vaginal Politics*) recently wrote in *Viva* magazine that she would choose to have one of these in preference to the possibility of error associated with a frozen biopsy as described above. However, office or needle biopsies are only suitable in some cases otherwise they too, can result in misdiagnosis — this time in the form of false negative.

## Hospitals

Besides surgeons, there are other specialists involved in the treatment of cancer, such as chemotherapists or radiotherapists. Ideally, decisions about the best way to treat a particular case should be made on the basis of joint discussion between all the relevant specialists, including the pathologist. However, this is by no means the general rule. In some hospitals, particularly the smaller ones, the surgeon may reign supreme, with the power to decide whether or not even to refer to a specialist from another discipline. It is best to go to the bigger hospitals with all the facilities.

Some of the bigger hospitals are better than others. Some doctors believe strongly that biologically active drugs should be used with early cases of breast cancer and not with just the more advanced cases. They believe that at the early stage of the disease the drugs are probably at their most effective. It is not the rule for these cytotoxic drugs to be used with early cases for two reasons. Firstly, their efficacy in these cases has not been proved conclusively, and secondly, experienced people are required in order to minimize the side effects of the drugs. Only centres with the capacity and above all, the time, are able to do this. The evidence is becoming increasingly strong, both in terms of survival and its quality, that this kind of chemotherapy should begin right at the start of treatment.

## TO SUM UP

There is of course much debate and research going on about treatment for breast cancer. As far as surgery is concerned, although figures now seem to show that less radical treatment is at least as effective in most cases, radical mastectomies do have their proponents, even in Britain. As far as accompanying treatment is concerned, this can range from hormone treatment (including possible removal of the ovaries), drugs to stimulate the body's defence mechanisms against the disease, drugs which kill off cells, and of course, radiotherapy. However, whatever is most suitable depends on a variety of factors; the kind, stage and place of the tumour, the age of the individual woman (particularly whether she is of childbearing age or past the menopause), and above all, the expertise of the technicians involved, their ability to treat each woman as an individual, and the resources available in the particular hospital. Some doctors, as an American surgeon has remarked, don't treat women, they treat themselves. In other words, they want to be able to feel that they have done everything they could for the patient — 'doing' being the operative word. Hence, the kinds of block-buster, major treatment programmes used especially in the USA, (eg.maximum surgery, maximum chemotherapy, maximum radiotherapy). Therefore if women are faced with breast cancer and want to know what the possibilities are, it is imperative that we should be in a position to ask for the objective opinions of at least two doctors with no particular axes to grind. Of course some people feel that they would rather not know what is happening but that should not mean that others should be prevented from knowing. People can be in a state of dire anxiety and fear simply because of a doctor's misguided belief that patients are being protected.

(This section consists of extracts from 3 articles by Jill Rakusen on breast cancer in *Spare Rib* Nos 37 and 42. For more information read these articles, and *Our Bodies, Ourselves*. See also ORGANIZATIONS and FURTHER READING.)

## CANCER OF THE CERVIX

This can be detected by looking at smears of cells from the neck of the womb but can also be found very early if you consult your doctor when you have unusual symptoms which *may* be signs of cancer:

Bleeding between periods.
Bleeding after intercourse.
Bleeding more than 6 months after the menopause.

## Erosion

Only 5 out of every 1000 women over 35 who have an erosion have cancer. An erosion is really just the inside lining of the womb which becomes visible at the opening of the neck of the womb (*cervical os*). The cells from inside are redder so it appears as a red patch. Most doctors will do a smear test if one is found. Pregnant women and women on the Pill have more erosions. This is due to hormonal changes and they often disappear by themselves.

## Smear Tests

Since the introduction of the cancer smear test, the age-related mortality of cervical cancer has fallen, though not as much as expected at first. Smears are called Pap smears after Dr Papanicolou, who first discovered that cancer cells are more sticky than ordinary cells and would stick to a wooden spatula if this was scraped around the neck of the womb.

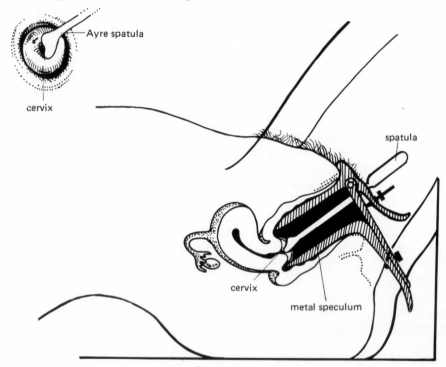

Pap smear test

Of all women found to have cervical cancer, 45 per cent survive the next 5 years. This includes many people in whom the cancer is far advanced before it is found, often because they are scared to go to their doctor for advice. It is very important to go to the doctor early should you have any abnormal bleeding, and to have regular smear tests. All women over 25 should have a smear test, ideally once every 2-3 years. However, because of time and money problems in the NHS, it is not able to provide this service for everyone, so every women should make sure she has at least 1 every 5 years. Whenever you have a pelvic examination, you should ask if a smear has been done and to know the result. Out of 1000 smears, 20 will be abnormal in some way, and only about 3 will show the changes of early cancer. Occasionally, cancer can appear suddenly in someone with a negative smear a few months before; but this is pretty rare. The smear may show several different 'abnormalities' which are not cancer, so don't be alarmed if you are asked to return for a further smear or treatment. For instance, there may be inflammatory changes due to an infection such as Thrush, which can be cleared up by simple treatment, but you should have a repeat smear after treatment.

*Suspicious or Abnormal Smears*
In these cases, odd or unusually large cells are seen on the smear. This may be a temporary change, or again it may be due to infection. However, changes like these may be signs of early cancer. You will be asked to have a repeat smear and if the changes are still there, you may be asked to go to hospital for a day or so. You will have a pelvic exam and the doctor may examine the cervix under anaesthetic. A ring-shaped piece of the edge of the cervix (where the smear was taken) may be removed. This is called a 'cone biopsy'. It is a minor procedure and although you may have slight pain the next day, it will not affect your sex life or ability to have children. If pre-cancerous changes are found, removing this piece will prevent cancer developing.

If cancer is revealed by smear or cone biopsy at an early stage, there is today almost 100 per cent likelihood of a cure if you have a hysterectomy. Usually the doctor will remove the ovaries at the same time; and X-ray treatment may be used as well. Results with this treatment are so good that I myself would not hesitate to undergo it. If you have cone biopsy you should make sure you are seen regularly every year for a smear, as very occasionally pre-cancerous cells may reappear and a repeat cone biopsy is necessary.

## CANCER OF THE UTERUS

This is less common than cancer of the cervix, and occurs mainly in women over 50. Smear tests are not often able to detect it. However, an early sign is bleeding long after the end of the menopause. If you have this symptom, your doctor should arrange for you to have a d&c (dilatation and curettage) under anaesthetic. The uterus is scraped, and the scrapings looked at under a microscope. Any cancer can be seen. Treatment is usually hysterectomy and X-ray therapy. 80 per cent of women who are treated early enough live for more than 5 years.

## CANCER OF THE VULVA

This is not very common and mainly occurs in women over 70. The first symptoms are an itchy vulva, or an ulcer on the edge of the vulva. In 99 per cent of cases, these symptoms will be due to a simple infection, but it's worth seeing a doctor as a simple operation could prevent an early cancer spreading.

## CANCER OF THE OVARY

This cancer is as common as cancer of the cervix, mainly in elderly people. 99 per cent of ovarian cysts are not cancerous, but merely sacs containing a fluid. Sadly, there is no way of diagnosing cancer of the ovary until symptoms such as pain start to occur. However, if you go for a smear test and have a pelvic examination, even just once every 5 years, the chances are that it would be found before it could cause too much trouble.

## FURTHER READING

*Breast Cancer, Self Examination: an aid to early detection* available from BUPA Medical Centre, Pentonville Rd, London N1 at 40p.

## ORGANIZATIONS

Women's National Cancer Control Campaign, 9 King Street, London WC2E 8HN: Tel 01-836 9901. Promotes extension of screening facilities and information.

The Mastectomy Association: Ms Betty Westgate, 1 Colworth Road, Croydon CRO 7 AD: Tel 01-654 8643.

British Cancer Council, 2 Harley Street, London W1: Tel 01-274 4002. Gives information.

National Society for Cancer Relief: Michael Sobell House, 30 Dorset Square, London NW1: Tel 01-723 6277.

Cancer Information Association, Gloucester Green, Oxford OE1 2EQ: Tel Oxford 46654.

Regional Cancer Services, in Leeds, Manchester, South West Thames and Wessex (contact local AHA or British Cancer Council for addresses). They provide an information and advisory service for anyone, including patients.

# WOMEN & MENTAL HEALTH

Mental health is as important as physical health. The two kinds of health are in fact so closely connected that they shouldn't be thought of separately or dealt with separately. When you're feeling lousy, it's often difficult to tell whether your problems have more to do with your mind, or with your body and where to begin to do something. Just as with physical health, your mental health can range from excellent to terrible. As with physical health, there are many more minor problems than major ones, and by dealing with the minor ones they are less likely to become major ones.

Serious mental health problems (often termed mental illnesses) affect more women than they do men, at least to the extent that more women come into contact with the mental health services (which are really concerned with mental illness and handicap) and they are more likely to spend some time as in-patients in a psychiatric hospital or unit. Women also take more *psychotropic drugs* (drugs which affect your blood such as tranquillizers, anti-depressants etc. and are more often diagnosied by their GPs as having 'mental health problems'. (This does not necessarily mean that women really do have more problems than men — it is only true to say they are defined this way more often.)

If you feel you have a mental health problem or somebody else feels they have, then treat it seriously. Before getting involved, here are some things to consider:

## Whose Problem Is It?

If you plan to do something about your own or help take on somebody else's, you will almost invariably find it's more complicated than you expected and takes more time. If you're taking on responsibility for seeing someone else through a difficult time, remember that letting them down or giving up because the going gets too tough and you can't handle it is *worse* than never having got involved in the first place.

## What About Very Serious Problems?

You can do something about a great many problems, but some are so serious you shouldn't tackle them. Whatever you think of the psychiatric services it's better to use them than to go under yourself, or to get you or others into a dangerous situation, or, usually, to take on the responsibility for preventing a serious suicide attempt. Almost everyone in an emotional crisis is afraid of losing control. They want to feel some kind of support and protection, and if you can't give that it's better not to try. A high proportion of those threatening suicide actually attempt it, and the greatest danger is not when energy is at its lowest, but when it is picking up a bit. Another indicator of seriousness is when very bizarre behaviour begins suddenly — then it is best to get medical help.

## What Kind of Support is Available?

If there's lots of strong support you'll have more chance of getting through when the going get's tough.

## Getting Better or Solving a Problem

This comes down to *doing* things that allow you or somebody else actually to gain more control over your own lives. Just talking about things or applying lots of intellectual theories or taking care of somebody so they don't have to do anything will prevent anything positive happening. Getting better also involves allowing yourself to feel things rather than just talking about them. Many times a good cry or burst of anger would be far better than hours of talking about why you feel that way.

## Problems are not Individual

They don't come about just because something is wrong with an individual. Physical and individual responses may be important, but also important are things like poverty, the kind of society people live in, and the way people's roles are defined. As is true of almost every kind of physical illness, for example, the rates of 'mental illness' are very much higher among poorer people. Thus mental health problems are also about politics.

Next it might be useful to look at some of the contrasts between healthy and unhealthy responses to life, and problems of living. This may be of help in identifying some problems.

1) Mentally healthy people feel problems can be worked on rather than that things are hopeless or that nothing is worth doing.

2) They can and do express a full range of emotions rather than just a few. (You're in trouble if you can't get angry or cry, for example.)

3) They have at least a few close friendships with people rather than none or only shallow ones.

4) They are realistic, rather than, for example, trying to be perfect or live up to an ideal or thinking they are worthless and terrible. They know everybody has strong and weak points.

5) They are problem-centred rather than self-centred, and more independent than dependent.

6) They need privacy and peace from time to time, rather than all the time or never.

7) They assume the basic responsibility for their own lives rather than playing the blaming game.

8) Their security comes from inside – not from manipulating or controlling others or setting themselves up to lose.

Here are some more specific signs of a lack of mental health. They become more serious as problems the more regularly they happen:

a) Not wanting to get up/do anything. Putting important things off.

b) Thinking everything is wonderful and possible.

c) Not trusting anyone, thinking everyone is hostile.

d) Not being able to concentrate, work at things, take care of self or other people or things.

e) Losing touch with needs, weaknesses, vulnerability; feeling you have to be perfect.

f) Emotions which seem to be uncontrolled or not at all approriate or out of proportion.

g) When the approach to problems becomes completely one-sided.

h) When 'crazy spaces' increase, or the reaction to them being touched is explosive. (We all have 'crazy spaces' and when somebody brings up these subjects or touches these spaces we react irrationally and out of proportion.)

i) When it's no longer possible to communicate effectively with the same people with whom it was formerly possible.

j) When a person's behaviour becomes self-destructive or destructive of others.

Everybody has these kinds of things happening to them to some degree and from time to time. You have to get a balance in assessing what is a normal reaction to your life and when your reactions are becoming a serious problem in your life. Before things get too serious, there are many things you can do to help yourself (or others).

*Do things that nurture yourself and take care of all of you.* It's important to eat well, something that you may not do, particularly when you get depressed. This means eating good food, with lots of fresh fruits and vegetables, enough protein etc. Eat regular, balanced meals rather than snacks in bits and pieces. The times when you have problems are the times when you need the *best* diet.

*You also need regular exercise,* and make it active and a bit exhausting. (This is also the time you need exercise the most and may feel least like getting it.) You can do set exercises or just some jumping and bending to a favourite record that makes you feel like moving. If you're really down, the first day or so will be hell — and it will take a good 3 or 4 days to feel the benefit. Try moving in ways or directions you're not used to. Stretch higher, curl up smaller, kick harder, move your head, legs, arms in the biggest possible circle. Exercise and movement often does a lot to move emotional states. Regular exercise will also make you feel more healthy, less tired and more optimistic.

*Give yourself some definite time and space in each day to do exactly what you want.* You might think of yourself as a loved child and then treat yourself as you would want to be treated.

*Give yourself a few treats.* You get more energy from the good things that happen to you. A treat might be just changing some small thing — clothes or a special food or something that would really please you.

*You need back-up and support.* The best support will come from the people who like you as you are, whom you can trust, whom you feel *comfortable* with. Start spending more time with people you feel comfortable with and less with the uncomfortable ones. It might help to draw a map of all the people you know, including your family. Put yourself in the middle, close friends and family next out, then not so close friends and family etc. Link up all the ones that know each other with lines. Put spiky lines around the ones that make you feel uncomfortable. Think about the links you could build on to get better support. think about links you could cut — some of the ones which make you uncomfortable.

*It's not very useful to think about changing into 'a better person' or to somebody who is mentally healthy.* It's more useful to accept yourself as you are right now as OK, including all the things you do that contradict each other and the feelings and actions that change from one moment to the next. You make real movement only from the base of knowing who you are now.

*Finding out who you really are is very difficult.* Almost all of us would rather pretend, or blame what happens on others, or live in the past or worry about the future at the expense of who we are now.

One thing that helps to get in touch with who you are now is to keep a diary about your feelings and reactions to things. This will also help to show some patterns in your thinking — do you always feel or describe yourself as a baddy for example? Be sure to notice the good things you've felt and done.

Every morning before you get up or at night before you go to sleep take a 5-minute tour around every part of the inside of your body. Notice which parts you feel good or bad about, which ones feel tense, tired, weak, strong. This will give you lots of clues about how you're really feeling and what you need to do for yourself each day.

If there's a special problem that's bothering you, instead of describing the problem, ask instead 'What's this sort of behaviour a solution to?'

This often helps to work a lot of things out.

Write a letter to somebody important to you – which you don't have to send – and tell them about their influence on you and write all the things you haven't been able to say.

*Just as was suggested with movement and exercise, increase the possibilities for extending your range of emotions.* Forget about trying to act 'grown-up' – it's harmful and useless. Do something about making more opportunity for fun, laughter, play and tenderness. This will give you more energy to get through the serious and heavy parts of life that everyone has to get through. You also need possibilities to express anger and aggression.

*Linked with this, have a campaign to put more time and energy into the positive – and less time and thinking into the 'poor me', masochistic bit.* This is linked with moving from just operating on a self-analyzing, individual level to a level where there is social potential as well. Your aim is to affect your world and to have more control over it. Gaining more control means getting involved with people and doing things rather than just thinking or talking about them.

*Get the idea of moving through things rather than around them or pretending they aren't there.* This means accepting and going through the hurt, rejection, grief or resentment rather than blaming, which is a cop-out. It's far better to cry it all out or to get angry and say it than to keep a stiff upper lip or be a martyr and just take it. You need to get through your feelings rather than deny them.

*Look at criticism – about you or somebody else.* This too often tends to be global and ends up as an attack on the person. Instead look at specific behaviour'– what you or another person do. Nobody is all bad or good; but you can like or dislike, feel comfortable or uncomfortable about some of the things they do. (See books on assertiveness training, in FURTHER READING.)

*Look at the issue of power.* It's very easy to look for answers outside yourself, yet if you expect to find the answers to your life outside yourself, it's an illusion. It's very easy to give your power away – eg. everybody else is wonderful, someone in particular has the answers to everything, here is someone who can make your whole life worthwhile etc. When you give your power away you can't make an impact on the world and you give up your responsibility.

*Look at the concept of guilt.* It's useless, self-destructive and a great immobilizer. Look for the resentments that may be behind the guilt. If you're feeling guilty about a mistake, then look at it as just a mistake which everybody makes and can do at least something about. Think also about early 'shoulds' and 'shouldn'ts' that were laid down when you were a child.

*Look at aggression and anger.* Many women 'learn' these feelings aren't OK and they often deny them. We all contain everything so look for your

99

malice and recognize that it's OK (You still have the choice of what you do about it — a straight statement that you're angry, banging away at a pillow, turning it back inside and sulking etc.).

If you're angry it means you have an investment. The real hurt is withdrawal, feeling hopeless about yourself and others.

*If you choose to attend some sort of group for support or to learn about yourself, make sure you trust the leader and that you feel comfortable about what part you are asked to play.* Make sure the leader, if there is one, is prepared to give you his/her telephone number and be contacted after the group in case you need support. (There are too many groups which rip you off both financially and emotionally.)

*If you choose to go to a doctor for either a physical or emotional problem (or you are unsure what your problem is):* consider keeping an accurate written record of what you are feeling — the 'symptoms'; take a friend with you if you can't face it alone. (The situation is usually that if you or your friend has some medical qualification or high status, you'll be taken more seriously.)

Drugs should only be used to help get you to a state where you can better deal with the underlying problems (where mental ill health is concerned). Even these aren't always much or any help. You can always ask to see another doctor or get a psychiatric opinion if you feel you aren't getting the help and consideration you need.

Sometimes it helps to 'role-play' your visit to the doctor with a friend beforehand. Remember that most doctors are middle class men and they will too often suggest you will feel better by fitting in more with the traditional 'woman's role'. Also, if you've ever been to your doctor with an 'emotional' problem, there is a tendency to think that any other problems you may then come with are also emotional. Here support and a record of 'symptoms' will help.

*If you or somebody else is feeling paranoid (persecuted, everybody's against you, ignoring you, after you etc.), it's almost always partly justified.* This feeling needs to be taken seriously. Look for the underlying oppressions.

*A lot of good comes from getting involved in doing things.* Doing things, especially the kinds you don't have to think about, often work to move your feeling and thinking. You can do many things without having to understand or explain why — make space for the ones which give you energy. And any action which will help to tackle problems is likely to make you feel better. For example, if you are a depressed mother with young children, it's better to get involved organizing a play-group or to get a part-time job than to spend the time feeling put upon and depressed. Despite the many myths around, your children will not be ruined if you are not always there. They will be better off with a happier mother.

*When you choose things to do, choose things that you are likely to succeed at.* You need success and to feel you can handle things. Thus it's better to make little steps at a time than big leaps. You don't need more failures or 'put-downs'.

*When you decide what you need and want, think about asking for it 100 per cent of the time.* People can't read your mind. Don't feel you don't deserve it. You are more likely to get it if you ask for it; if you can't get it it's because the other person doesn't want or can't give it to you, not because you don't deserve it. When you can ask for what you want, you are better able to give others what they want and need. This benefits everybody.

These suggestions are for problems, either your own or other people's, that you feel you can cope with. If you feel you *can't* cope with a mental health problem, find out from the address below, your doctor if he/she is sympathetic, or a health group, where you should go for the best medical help.

## FURTHER READING

*Medicines*, Peter Parish (Penguin 1976); information about tranquillizers, stimulants, anti-depressants as well as other drugs.

*Conjoint Family Therapy*, Virginia Satir (Science and Behaviour Books, Inc 1967)

*Born to Win*, Muriel James and Dorothy Jongeward (Business Services 1971); on Transactional Analysis.

*The Assertive Woman*, Stanlee Phelps and Nancy Austin (Impact Pubs 1975)

*When I Say No I Feel Guilty*, Manuel J. Smith (Bantam 1975), both on assertiveness training.

*Getting Clear (Bodywork for Women)*, Anne Kent Rush (Wildwood House 1974)

*Women and Madness*, Phyllis Chesler (Allen Lane 1974)

*Complaints and Disorders: the Sexual Politics of Sickness*, Barbara Ehrenreich and Deirdre English (Writers and Readers Publishing Cooperative 1976)

*Not Made of Wood*, Jan Foudraine (Quartet 1974)

*Readings in Radical Psychiatry*, ed Claude Steiner (Grove Press 1972); good on the politics of psychiatry and on women.

*The Barefoot Psychoanalyist Book 1*, compiled by John Southgate and Rosemary Randall (The Association of Karen Horney Psychoanalytic Counsellors); an illustrated book about an approach to co-counselling or reciprocal counselling.

*Be The Person You Were Meant To Be*, Dr Jerry Greenwald (Dell 1973); an easy to understand and practical approach to problems based on Gestalt Theory.

## ORGANIZATIONS

If you have practical problems, questions about legal rights, or want advice about mental health problems, one place you can contact is MIND (National Association for Mental Health), 22 Harley Street, London W1N 2ED: Tel 01-637 0741.

# DRUGS

Drugs originally came from plant, animal and mineral sources, but nowadays they are mostly synthetic. They come in many forms: as tablets, capsules, injections, mixtures, ointments, sprays ...

## Tablets

Tablets are just highly compressed powder. They act more slowly than injections (unless they are the type that you keep under your tongue, rather than swallow, in which case they are absorbed into the bloodstream quickly). Tablets are very convenient to take but sometimes irritate your stomach (eg.aspirin). Sometimes they don't break up easily and then they don't get absorbed properly, so it is often useful to break or crush them in your mouth first before swallowing (eg. with non-soluble aspirin) unless instructed otherwise.

## Capsules

Capsules are powder or granules in a gelatine case that is specifically designed to break up beyond your stomach where the drug will be well absorbed. Always swallow them whole.

## Mixtures

Mixtures are often used to disguise nasty-tasting drugs (eg. Noctec for sleeping), or for children's medicines, or for drugs which would go soggy if made into tablets.

## Injections

Injections are given if the drugs have to get into your bloodstream as quickly as possible to take quick effect, or if a drug would be destroyed by passing through your stomach (eg. insulin, benzyl-penicillin).

## Locally Applied Drugs

Locally applied drugs (eg.skin ointments, vaginal pessaries, inhaler aerosol sprays) are designed to get the drug where it is most needed and not elsewhere, so that you can take smaller doses and minimize side effects.

You should take drugs in the dose and at the times stated in the instructions:

*Take no more and no less* than the prescribed or recommended dose. Too little means ineffective amounts of the drug in your body (especially dangerous with antibiotics). Too much can also be dangerous and give you more side effects, especially with children. Smaller bodies need less drug; and the very young have immature livers and kidneys which cannot get rid of drugs as well as an adult's can.

*Take drugs at the correct times.* A tablet to be taken 3 times a day is destroyed by your liver or excreted by your kidneys quite fast, so in order to keep effective blood levels of the drug all day it is no good taking all 3 at once and hoping that is the same thing. Drugs destroyed more slowly can be taken less often. Instructions to take drugs at meal times are often just for your convenience in remembering; but some must be taken before meals so that they are quickly and regularly absorbed from an empty stomach. Others should be taken after meals because they would irritate an empty stomach.

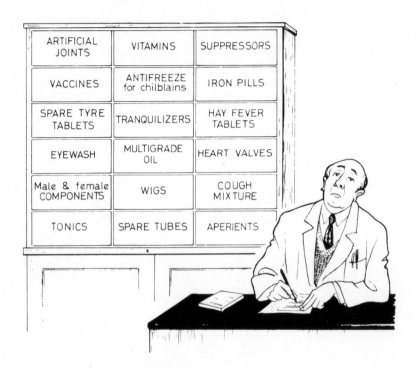

## PAINKILLERS (ANALGESICS)

Aspirin is generally the most effective over-the-counter drug. It reduces pain, fever and inflammation if taken in the right dose (adults, 2 x 300 mg tablets every 4 hours). Soluble aspirin is preferable, cheap brands being just as good as expensive ones. Aspirin is an irritant and may cause bleeding in your stomach, so do not use for hangovers, if you are feeling sick, or if you have ulcers or are taking anticoagulants (to prevent blood clots), or if you are elderly (blood loss may cause vitamin C deficiency).

Children are very susceptible to aspirin poisoning, so never give more than the recommended children's dose, and keep bottles of aspirin locked up.

If you cannot take aspirin, paracetamol is the next best thing. It does not irritate your stomach, but overdoses do damage your liver. It has no anti-inflammatory action. Both aspirin and paracetamol act locally at the site of pain.

Most other analgesics are on prescription only because they are addictive drugs like morphine, codeine and methadone. They have a more powerful action than aspirin or paracetamol, and act on your brain, rather than on the site of your pain. Often they make you feel happier too, so that you forget your pain.

## MINOR TRANQUILLIZERS

These act mainly on your spinal cord, to dampen down your reactions and relax your muscles, so reducing anxiety. Examples are Librium, Valium and Miltown. They are rarely addictive in the way that, for example, morphine is; but you can get psychologically dependent on them if you take them for a long time. Your reactions will be slowed down, so beware when driving. Avoid alcohol, or you will get very sleepy: and never drive if you have taken these drugs in conjunction with alcohol. They are not very good for the elderly, who can get drowsy and confused if they take these drugs. Other side effects are dry mouth, headache and blurred vision.

## MAJOR TRANQUILLIZERS

These act mainly on areas of the brain involved in emotions and wakefulness. Examples are Amargyl, Chloractil, Largactil, Protamyl, Melleril, Motiden, Motival, Serenace and Stelazine. They are used to treat anxiety and tension, schizophrenia and other major mental illnesses. They also prevent sickness. Avoid taking alcohol or barbiturate with major tranquillizers, as the combination may make you unconscious.

## ANTIDEPRESSANTS

These act to increase the amounts of natural chemicals in your brain, which are assumed to drop below normal in some types of depression, bringing about a change of mood. However, not all types of depression are helped by these drugs and it is not known why; nor is it possible to predict very well who will respond to these drugs and who won't. They take effect only after 1 to 6 weeks. There are 2 basic types of antidepressant drugs:

**Mono-Amine Oxidase Inhibitors**

(eg. Actomol, Marplan, Marsilid, Niamid, Parnate) must not be taken with certain foods such as Bovril, Marmite, cheese, broad beans, yogurt, strong beers or wines, or with over-the-counter cold cures such as Procol or Contac. In conjunction with these substances, the drugs could raise your blood pressure, causing headaches or more serious side effects. They should also not be taken with other drugs available on prescription such as barbiturates, amphetamines or the other type of antidepressants (see below).

Your doctor should warn you about all these things.

## Tricyclic Antidepressants

(eg. Berkomine, Dimipressin, Ethipram, Laroxyl, Limbritol, Petrofran, Saroten, Tofranil, Triptafen, Tryptizol) must not be taken with alcohol, drugs to reduce blood pressure, sleeping tablets or the other type of anti-depressants (see above); or with some local anaesthetics (so warn your dentist). These drugs are also used for treating bedwetting in children.

## SLEEPING TABLETS

Barbiturates (Amytal, Nembutal, Protamyl, Rapidal, Seconal, Sonergan, Soneryl, Tuinal) generally damp down your brain activity. They are very dangerous with alcohol which also damps down your brain activity. They are addictive if taken for long periods. Other potentially addictive types of sleeping tablets are Mandrax, Meseldin, Paldona, Revonal, Welldorm. Obviously, if taken for a short while to get you over a bad patch, they cause no harm, but if taken for months they will be addictive. Many doctors now prescribe Mogadon (a stronger form of Valium) which is much less addictive. Avoid alcohol and antihistamines (which are contained, for instance, in travel-sickness pills) with all these types of sleeping tablet. These drugs may make elderly people confused.

## ANTIBIOTICS

These are too numerous to list! They kill bacteria or enable your body's natural defences to kill them, but rarely kill viruses (so are no good for the common cold). Doctors prescribe far too many antibiotics for trivial illnesses that would get better by themselves (eg. just by keeping warm in bed for a day or so): so question your doctor whether they are really necessary for you. If they are, it is very important to take the right dose and complete the whole course of drugs, otherwise resistant organisms will start to grow, and you will end up with a worse infection than the one you started with.

Antibiotics can be divided roughly into 2 types: broad spectrum and narrow spectrum. Broad spectrum drugs combat many different types of organism (eg. the tetracyclines like Achromycin, Aureomycin, Berkmycen, Clinimycin, and the orally-taken penicillins like Ampiclox, Magnapen, Penbritin, Talpen). Side effects are common; rashes with the penicillins; nausea and diarrhoea, and Thrush overgrowth in the throat and vagina with the tetracyclines. Tetracyclines also affect bone and teeth development, so should never be taken after the fifth month of pregnancy and should not be taken by children under 8 years of age as it stains their teeth. Tetracyclines should also not be taken in conjunction with iron tablets or milk, because they do not get absorbed if iron or calcium is present. Penicillin (given usually by injection) is somewhere between broad and narrow spectrum in its action. Allergic reactions to penicillin of all types are not uncommon, and you should warn doctors and dentists if you know you are sensitive. Narrow spectrum antibiotics are active against only a few organisms (eg. Nystatin and Nystan specifically combat Thrush). When taking Flagyl for Trichomonas infection of the vagina, avoid alcohol or you will be sick; don't take the very short, high-dose courses if you're pregnant; and make sure your partner is treated too.

## FURTHER READING

*Take a Pill – the Drug Industry: Private or Public?* ( Marxists in Medicine 20p)

## USEFUL SOURCES OF INFORMATION

(MIMS) Monthly Index of Medical Specialities. Ask your doctor for an old copy. It is brief but tells you what chemicals are in which drug, what the drug is for, and some of the side effects and contra-indications.

Any book on drugs in the medical section of your library: but you will often need a medical dictionary too, in order to decipher the jargon. Rewarding if you like detective work.

## ORGANIZATIONS

Pharmacists are a very much underrated, under-used source of information. They often know more about the drugs you are taking than your doctor does.

Mental Patients Union. They have produced a directory of the side effects of psychiatric drugs: obtainable from MPU, Robin Farquarson House, 37 Mayola Road, London E5. 25p plus postage.

# NUTRITION

Good nutrition is an important aspect of self help. If you are susceptible to disease it is because your natural resistance is low. Lowered resistance comes partially from imbalances in the body, largely vitamin and mineral excesses and deficiencies. Though factors such as stress can cause these imbalances, good nutrition can do a lot to offset damaging effects; diet alone has an enormous effect on the individual's susceptibility to disease. Diseases as diverse as dental decay, colitis, heart disease and some forms of cancer have been linked with dietary imbalances of various kinds.

Nutrition is a very complex subject and it must be remembered that every individual has different food requirements. Nevertheless there are some basic principles for both vegetarians and meat eaters. (Obviously our eating habits are also constrained by our jobs, our kids, other people we live with etc.)

1) Eat only when you're hungry. Any food we eat the body has to deal with. It takes energy to digest food and if we eat more food than we require (common in Britain, especially particular types of food such as sugar), then an excessive amount of the body's energies will be needed for digestion. As a result the digestive processes will become less efficient and the body may become clogged by waste products that it no longer has the energy to get rid of. *Over-eating* may lead to obesity, which does itself predispose to a wide range of diseases.

2) Eat foods that are in as natural a form as possible. Avoid refined and processed foods such as sugar (especially white), white flour products, white rice and all tinned foods. In processing, the chemical constituents of food are changed, many nutrients being destroyed by heating and by the addition of chemical preservatives etc. Whenever possible eat fruit and vegetables which are grown without chemical fertilizers as these alter the natural mineral balance of the food. Similarly, avoid battery-fed poultry and hormonally fattened beef and pork. If you are eating well, vitamin tablets should be unnecessary, and they are no substitute for natural food.

3) Eat some protein (meat, eggs, cheese, nuts, beans, brown rice) every day and include in your diet as much fresh fruit and vegetables as possible, preferably raw. If possible, grow your own vegetables.

4) Learn how to cook food so as to preserve as much nutritional value as possible — it is especially important not to overcook vegetables, since much of the nutritional value is then lost in the water.

## FOOD CO-OPS

Most health food stores are a rip-off so if you want to start eating healthily they're not a good place to begin. Bulk buying reduces food costs considerably. All you require to start a food co-op is a group of interested people, one of whom has the use of a car to go to the local market once a week and buy fruit and vegetables by the case. Unless you're living in the middle of a city you can often arrange to buy food from a local farmer – poultry, cheese, eggs etc. Foods like cereals, nuts, oils etc. may be more difficult, though this is less and less the case. In London the Bulk Food Store in Prince of Wales Crescent, NW1, sells bulk brown rice, soy sauce, honey, oil and many other items at around half the retail price. This co-op works in conjunction with other bulk food stores throughout Britain and has a list of food co-ops in all parts of the country. Write for information about food co-ops in your area.

A women's group can easily start a co-op together, or you could put ads in local shops or the local paper to find other interested people. A food co-op takes a little time but can save a lot of money and be the start of a change to a healthier diet.

## FURTHER READING

*Diet for a Small Plant*, Frances Moore Lappe (Ballantine 1975)

*Our Bodies, Ourselves*, ed Angela Phillips and Jill Rakusen (Penguin 1978)

# SMOKING

Much smoking advertising in this country and the USA is linked to ideas
of liberation. During and after the Second World War women began to
smoke a lot, joining in with the men. Now over 30 per cent of adult
women smoke, and many begin at school at the age of 12 or less. In 1970,
12 per cent of 12-18 year olds smoked. Studies in Europe, USA and Japan
show that smokers spend 15 days more a year sick in bed than non-
smokers.

## RISKS

### Cancers

1) lung: smoking over 40 cigarettes a day increases the risk 30 times.
Lung cancer is now the second most common cancer in women — the incidence has tripled in one generation. 10 years after stopping the risk falls to
non-smokers levels. It is often thought that cigars and pipes carry no risk
but the risk is only slightly less. Not inhaling lessens but does not abolish
the risk. Now 1 in 9 men over 45 die from lung cancer and women are
approaching this figure. Signs to look for are coughing blood, loss of
weight and appetite and a sudden distaste for cigarettes. It is not always
too late.

2) Mouth and throat cancer: smoking predisposes to this.

3) Bladder cancer: a substance known to be inhaled in cigarette smoke,
napthylamine, predisposes to cancer. Smokers have a higher incidence of
bladder cancer.

### Bronchitis and Emphysema

There are 3 times the number of cases in smokers. Smoke impairs the
ability of the bronchial cells to deal with infection and destroys the hairs
that waft dirt up out of the lungs. It also increases the secretion of mucus
in the air passages.

### Strokes

In women of 45-55 who smoke the incidence of strokes and heart disease
is doubled.

### Pregnancy

Infertility is increased in smokers. Smokers have smaller babies and an
increased incidence of stillbirths and babies dying in early life. This is
thought to be due to a decrease in the blood flow to the baby — as much
as 40 per cent less.

## Peptic (stomach or duodenal) Ulcer

There is a 50 per cent higher rate of these in smokers. Stopping is the only thing apart from bed rest known to help healing of ulcers. Also, nicotine is an irritant to the lining of the stomach.

## Gum Disease

This is debatable, but may be made worse by smoke.

Many women fear they'll put on weight if they stop — but this is only because food tastes better. If you don't eat more you won't gain weight. Happily the overall consumption of cigarettes is starting to decrease, but anti-smoking campaigns will get nowhere as long as cigarette companies make huge profits out of us suckers.

# THE NATIONAL HEALTH SERVICE

The National Health Service (NHS) was introduced by the post-war Labour Government in 1948 with the intention of giving everyone – regardless of their means – free and equal access to all medical services at the time of need. Although it attracted much international interest as the first 'socialized' health system in the Western world, most European countries have now established their own medical insurance schemes. These countries have also invested significantly more money in health care than Britain, and we have fewer doctors and dentists for our population size than they do.

In fact, Britain spends less than 5 per cent of her Gross National Product on health (less, for example, than on defence). Consequently, despite the high salaries and special privileges demanded by the consultants, most of our 800,000 health service workers are grossly overworked and underpaid. As patients, we are conscious of antiquated hospital buildings and long waiting lists, but the continuing inequalities in medical provision between regions and social classes are less well known.

## WHO RUNS THE NHS?

After 26 years of administrative chaos the NHS reorganization of 1974 has at least succeeded in unifying and co-ordinating the hospitals, local authority health services, and the family doctors to provide an interlocking system. Unfortunately – for us, the patients – it has also created an even more hierarchical management structure. In the past we had *some* representation at all managerial levels, but now 'management ability will be the main criterion for the selection of members' of health authorities. Simultaneously, the interest of the health professions (but no manual workers in the service) have been safeguarded even more vigorously in the reorganized NHS. Doctors, dentists, nurses etc not only have members on the Regional and Area Health Authorities, but also have professional advisory committees at all levels which the Authorities have a duty to consult. More important still, the way in which doctors have now been integrated into the managerial machinery at district level allows them an effective veto power over management decisions.

## WHAT SAY DO WE HAVE AS PATIENTS?

Very little. Successive governments have been so nervous of challenging doctors' professional claims for fear of losing their collaboration in the

NHS, that patients' interests have been overridden in an effort to appease the medical profession. The only outlet for the 'consumer's voice' in the reorganized NHS is the Community Health Council (CHC) in each district. The CHC membership of 18-30 people (serving a population of tens or even hundred of thousands) is not elected by anyone, but largely appointed by local authorities and the Regional Health Authority, with one third of the members being nominated by local voluntary bodies. Although women's groups, community groups and militant pressure groups may qualify as 'voluntary bodies', they are the organizations least likely to get the small number of CHC places because priority tends to go to established service organizations for the old, handicapped, blind etc, and to church bodies, Red Cross etc. Once on the CHC, members serve for 4 years, but they may be re-appointed and serve for up to 8!

But don't worry — the CHC has no legal power or responsibility anyway. Its members can inspect health service institutions and advise complainants of the procedures to follow, and it reports annually to the Area Health Authority. These advisory and watchdog functions are no substitute for effective patient participation but it may still be a good idea to try and get a representative from local women's groups on to the CHC to fight for women's health interests. For instance, Archway Women's Liberation Group already has a member on Islington CHC in London; and there are probably other examples. And remember that members of the public can also attend CHC meetings (which should allow questions and comments), so try going along. Phone your local Town Hall for details.

## HOW DO WE PAY FOR THE NHS?

The National Insurance contributions deducted from our wage packets only account for 10 per cent of all health service costs, while charges for prescriptions, dental treatment etc only cover a further 5 per cent. In fact, the great bulk of NHS expenditure is met from our ordinary taxes. So although we get 'free' medical treatment when we need it, we are certainly paying for the privilege!

## HOW TO CHANGE YOUR DOCTOR

### If You Move

Don't wait until you need treatment to find a new doctor. The local Family Practitioner Committee produces a list of all NHS doctors in the area. You'll find its address under 'National Health Service' in the phone book (in old directories it may appear as 'Executive Council' instead of 'Family Practitioner Committee', but it's the same thing). Lists of doctors are sometimes available in main post offices and public libraries too.

A doctor can refuse to accept you as a patient, without giving a reason, unless you need immediate treatment. And if the doctor does treat you in these circumstances, it doesn't mean you have been accepted as a patient.

When you've found a doctor, you both fill in the appropriate sections on your medical card, and the doctor sends it to the local Family Practitioner Committee. You will get a new medical card and your new doctor will be sent your medical records. If you change your address, but wish to keep the same doctor, you have to tell him your new address and make sure he'll continue to treat you. If you can't find a doctor who'll accept you, apply to your local Family Practitioner Committee – they will allocate you to one if necessary. This also applies if you are dissatisfied or away from home.

**If You Are Dissatisfied**

If you don't get on with your doctor, you can change him/her – but it's not always easy and you may have to be very persistent. The doctor you want may be too busy or anxious not to 'poach' a colleague's patients. But if you find a new doctor, there are 2 systems for changing:

1) If your present doctor agrees to the change, your old doctor, your new one and you sign your medical card. It is then sent to the local Family Practitioner Committee and you will get a new card in due course.

2) If you don't want to tell your present doctor, send your medical card to your local Family Practitioner Committee saying you want to transfer – you don't have to give a reason. Your card will be returned with a form in it. Fill in part of this form and send it and your medical card to the doctor you want to transfer to (you should already have found out if he/she'll have you). She/he fills in the rest of the form – you are then on his/her list. You will eventually get a new medical card. Until you're actually on the new doctor's list you can carry on being treated by your old doctor. He/she won't know about your application for transfer. (Incidentally, your doctor is entitled to take you off her/his list if she/he wants.)

**If You Are Away From Home**

If you need treatment while away from home for 3 months or less, you can apply to any NHS doctor. He/she need not accept you unless it's an emergency. If accepted, you become a temporary patient. If you're staying in an area for more than 3 months, register with a doctor permanently.

**In General**

Doctors are not allowed to advertise and no list will tell you anything except their qualifications and occasionally special interests in pregnancy or children etc. To find a non-sexist doctor is obviously difficult and can really be done only through personal recommendations – perhaps women's groups could try and compile their own information about sympathetic GPs and those to avoid at all costs! It would be very useful to any woman new to an area to be able to contact a local women's group and be given this kind of help.

## HOW TO COMPLAIN

### About Your GP

(Or your dentist, optician, chemist ...) The existing complaints machinery just doesn't consider the sort of things people tend to be most dissatisfied about: waiting, surgery hours and the attitudes of doctors. A 'legitimate' complaint would deal only with a doctor's *clinical* negligence – eg. if he/she hasn't sent you to a specialist you thought you needed; or not visited you at home when you felt sure it was necessary.

It is important to complain in writing within *8 weeks* to the Clerk of your Family Practitioner Committee (in phone book under 'National Health Service'). They will investigate your complaint and perhaps hold a private hearing with both sides present. If your complaint is considered justified, money will be withheld from the doctor's pay (usually about £100). However, you will get nothing unless you take the doctor to court – and few people have the time and money to do this. If the Family Practitioner Committee decides against you, you can appeal against the decision to the Secretary of State. If you wanted to do this, it would be a good idea to enlist the help of your local MP. If your complaint is about the doctor's misconduct – breach of confidence or sexual assault, for example – you must complain to the General Medical Council in London.

### About Your Hospital Treatment

Believe it or not, there is no statutory machinery for hospital complaints, and despite the government's 'request' that hospitals should include information about complaints procedures in their admission booklets, few of them do so. Given the uncertainty of this situation, it would be in your own interests to try and resolve the problem at as low a level as possible: with your consultant or the ward sister, for example. If this fails, or you feel your problem warrants fuller investigation, write to the District Administrator c/o the hospital concerned. It would also be a good idea to contact the local Community Health Council and inform them of your complaint – they cannot investigate it themselves, but should advise you of what action to take. Also, the CHC should know what difficulties people are having in their local hospitals. There may be occasions when legal action is appropriate, but hospitals tend to take the attitude that you should either sue or shut up, so don't be pushed into court action unless it's something pretty drastic. If you are taking legal action, your solicitor should contact The British Academy of Forensic Sciences, Department of Forensic Medicine, London Hospital Medical College, Turner Street, London E1. They will provide an 'expert witness' to give a clinical assessment of the situation.

## The Health Service Commissioner

Although he can be approached directly by members of the public, he can only investigate complaints which have first been before the relevant Area Health Authority and for some reason have not been resolved. But the Commissioner cannot deal with complaints about GPs, cannot investigate any matters of clinical judgment, and cannot consider complaints which could — even in theory — be brought before a court of law.

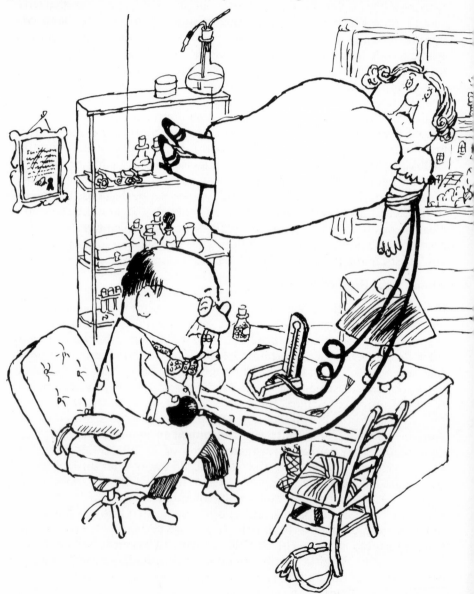

Given these absurd limitations, it isn't surprising that the Commissioner finds the big majority of patients' grievances outside his jurisdiction. In effect, all he can investigate are administrative and organizational complaints!

## HELP WITH MEDICAL COSTS

### Free prescriptions

The current charge for each item prescribed by a doctor is 20p. However, if you are in any of the categories below, you are entitled to free prescriptions:

1) Children under 16; women 60 or over; men 65 or over. Just complete a declaration on the back of your prescription before handing it to the chemist.

2) Expectant mothers. Use form FW8 from your doctor, health visitor or midwife to apply for an *exemption certificate* (see note below).

3) Women who have had a child in the last 12 months; people suffering from certain medical conditions, eg. diabetes — see Department of Health and Social Security (DHSS) leaflet FP91/EC91 for list of conditions. Use form FP91/EC91, from your local social security office or post office, to apply for an exemption certificate (see note below).

4) People already getting supplementary benefit or family income supplement. You should automatically get an authorization form so that you can apply for an exemption certificate (see below).

5) People with low incomes. Use form PC11 from your local social security office to apply for an exemption certificate (see below).

NB: If you apply for an *exemption certificate* for any of the above reasons, you may have to pay for prescriptions until you receive the certificate. In this case, make sure you ask the chemist for receipt form EC57. Use this, with the exemption certificate, to get a refund at the post office later.

### Free or Reduced Dental Charges

Charges for NHS dental treatment are at half the actual cost up to a maximum of £3.50 per course of treatment. Exemptions are as follows:

1) Children and young people under 21; expectant mothers; women who have had a child in the last 12 months. Just sign a declaration on the dentist's *treatment form*.

2) People already getting supplementary benefit, family income supplement, free prescriptions, or free milk and vitamins because of low income. Ask your dentist for form F1D, complete it and send it to your local social security office.

3) People with low incomes. You may be eligible for free treatment, or some help towards the cost. Get form F11 from your local social security office, *and* form F1D from your dentist. Complete them and send them both to your social security office.

NB: All those qualifying for free/reduced dental charges should be entitled to similar help with optical charges; *except* for expectant mothers and women who have had a baby in the last 12 months. Ask your optician for details and the appropriate forms.

## FURTHER READING

*You and the National Health Service*, George Teeling Smith (Arrow Books and Health Education Council 1975)

*The Changing NHS*, R G S Brown (Routledge 1973)

*The Hazards of Work: How to Fight Them*, Patrick Kinnersley (Pluto Press 1974)

## ORGANIZATIONS

If you are in any doubt about your rights as a patient, or want help with a particular problem or complaint, try contacting The Patients Association, 335 Gray's Inn Road, London WC1X 8PX: Tel 01-837 7241. They also publish useful leaflets which you could ask your local library to stock. Remember, too, that you can obtain information and advice from your local Community Health Council: get its address from your library.

# SOCIAL SECURITY & SUPPLEMENTARY BENEFITS

If you or someone in your family is ill, then you or your family may be entitled to some form of support from the Department of Health and Social Security (DHSS) or the Supplementary Benefits Commission (SBC). However, the system is very complicated and depends on individual circumstances, so we can only outline the benefits to which you *may* be entitled, and then give information as to how you go about clarifying your own position, and making sure you get your own rights.

## NATIONAL INSURANCE

The basic idea of National Insurance is that you pay stamps while you are working and then you get money to live on while you are *not* working: if you are ill, having a baby, retired or just unemployed. For women, the system is particularly complicated, as women are treated differently from the point of view of paying for stamps and of getting benefits, depending on whether or not they are married. A single woman, if she is working, pays a stamp and claims benefit in the same way as a man. A married woman, however, is assumed to be dependent on her husband and she is thus given 3 choices: if she is not working, she may choose to pay no stamp at all (and thus be *totally* dependent on her husband's stamp for any benefits she ever needs); if she is working, she may choose to pay either a single woman's stamp or a married woman's stamp. The latter is much cheaper, but will not entitle her to the same benefits. (The married woman's stamp will eventually be phased out.) We shall briefly outline here those benefits which are likely to be payable in case of sickness and/ or maternity, but again we must emphasize the complexity of the scheme, and the necessity of following up our information for yourself by looking at some of the more detailed books and pamphlets listed at the end.

### Sickness

1) Single women. They get sickness benefit at the normal rate, if they have paid the required number of stamps.

2) Married women. If a married woman gets sick and she has not been working, then she is not entitled to any benefit at all. If her husband gets sick however, he can claim sickness benefit for himself plus a special

allowance for his wife as a dependant. If a married woman who is working gets sick and she has been paying the married woman's stamp only, then again she is not entitled to benefit.

If a married woman gets sick and she has been working and also paying the full ('single woman's') stamp, then she is entitled to sickness benefit, provided she has paid enough stamps in the previous contribution year. However, she is paid at a lower rate of benefit than a single woman or man, even though she has paid the same amount for her stamps. She is also prevented from claiming for her husband as a dependant, unless he is a permanent invalid.

Sickness benefit, at whatever rate, is payable for the first 28 weeks of any period of sickness, and to claim it you need to get a certificate from your doctor and send it to your local Social Security Office within 6 days of becoming too ill to work. After 28 weeks you can claim invalidity benefit if you are still too ill to work, and if you have paid the requisite number of contributions.

If you are single or married, but paying the full stamp, you may be entitled to an earnings related supplement to your sickness benefit, depending on how much you earned in the previous tax year. You do not need to make a special claim for this, but you should check to see if you are eligible, and if so whether it is being paid.

If you are injured at work, or get what is called a 'prescribed industrial disease', you may be entitled to industrial injuries benefit.

**Pregnancy**

There are 2 types of benefit available under the National Insurance Scheme for pregnant women, and these are *Maternity Grant* and *Maternity Benefit*.

The *Maternity Grant* is a lump sum of £25 which is payable whether you are single or married. If you are single then you must have paid or been credited with the required number of stamps in the previous contribution year before the baby is born. If you are married however, you may claim on either your own or your husband's contributions.

To claim, get form BM4 from your local Social Security Office or maternity or child welfare clinic. You can claim at any time from 9 weeks before the baby is due, to 3 months after it is born.

The *Maternity Allowance* is a weekly allowance normally payable for 11 weeks before the baby is born and for 7 weeks after the birth. You can claim it whether you are single or married, but you can only claim it on your *own* insurance and therefore you must have the required number of stamps in the year before the baby is born (for details see form N1 17A from DHSS).

You can only get maternity allowance when you have *stopped* paid employment, and to get the allowance fill in form BM4 as described above for maternity grant. You *must* claim between the beginning of the 14th week and the 11th week before the baby is due.

NB: (i) You *may* get earnings related supplement as with sickness benefit. (ii) You are not entitled to maternity benefits if you are under 16. (If you are under 16 and need help – financial or otherwise, contact the National Council for One Parent Families, 255 Kentish Town Road, London NW5: Tel 01-267 1361).

If you disagree with any decision made about your right to a National Insurance benefit you can appeal to the N I Tribunal. For details on how to do this, see Coote & Gill, or contact the Child Poverty Action Group (see below).

## Supplementary Benefit

If you find you need money to live on during sickness or pregnancy (or any other time) you may claim Supplementary Benefit. Your rights under this scheme are even more complicated than under the NI scheme, but basically your benefit is calculated by working out the basic allowance you and your dependants are entitled to, and there are fixed rates laid down for this. This is then added to the amount necessary to cover your rent and rates (unless the SBC officer thinks these are unreasonably high) and any additional allowance you may claim if you have 'exceptional needs' (special food, heavy laundry expenses for example). The total of these 3 items is what you are entitled to. However, most of the income you have is then subtracted from this amount you are entitled to, and what remains is what you are actually paid.

NB: (i) You cannot claim SB if you are married and living with your husband (he must claim for you). (ii) If you are single and claim SB while living with a man you may be caught by the 'cohabitation rule' which assumes him to be financially responsible for you and therefore leads to your benefit being cut off.

If you are unhappy about any decision made by the SBC, you can appeal to the SB Tribunal. For details see under National Insurance.

## FURTHER READING

*Women's Rights: A Practical Guide*, Anna Coote and Tess Gill (2nd edition, Penguin 1977)

*National Welfare Benefits Handbook*, Child Poverty Action Group 1972, available from CPAG, 1 Macklin Street, London WC2

*The Penguin Guide to Supplementary Benefits*, Tony Lynes (Penguin 1972)

## ORGANIZATIONS

For further help contact your local claimants' union. If you cannot find out whether one exists you could try and get information from SE London Claimants' Union, The Albany, Creek Road, London SE8: Tel 01-692 1047. You can also contact the Citizen's Rights Office at the CPAG address above or phone them at 01-405 5942. They are especially good in helping with specific claims and will represent you at tribunals.

# INFORMATION & ADDRESSES

A list of health groups can go out of date very quickly, so we suggest you contact your nearest women's liberation group and ask if there is a health group or anyone interested in starting one with you. To find out where your nearest women's group is, contact WIRES (Women's Information Referral and Enquiry Service). Send a stamped addressed envelope to WIRES, c/o 30 Blenheim Terrace, Leeds 2: Tel: Leeds 35561.

## OTHER USEFUL ORGANIZATIONS

Release, 1 Elgin Avenue, London W9: Tel: 01-289 1123. Emergency number for outside office hours: 01-603 8654. Women coming to Release can get help and advice on their legal and welfare rights and they are able to call on the help of reliable solicitors whenever necessary. Pregnancy counselling figures as a major part of the work and help with abortion (both through the National Health and the private sector), contraception and sterilization is also given.

Rape Counselling and Research Centre, PO Box 42, London N6 5BU: Tel: 01-340 6913. 24 hr. emergency number is 01-340 6145.

## SUBSCRIBE TO:

*Women's Abortion and Contraception Campaign Newsletter.* Send 50p for 3 issues, including postage, to: Bristol WACC, 11 Waverley Road, Bristol BS0 6ES.

*Women's Report* has a health section in each issue with latest news presented from a feminist viewpoint. Subscription £2.00. Send cheques and postal orders to Women's Report, 14 Aberdeen Road, Wealdstone, Harrow, Middlesex.

*Spare Rib* has occasional health articles — you can order back issues too from Spare Rib, 27 Clerkenwell Close, London EC1. 1 year's subscription £4.44.

*WIRES* puts out a newsletter twice a month. Individual subscription is £5.00 a year — £3.00 if you're very poor.

## USEFUL BOOKSHOPS

We think it is useful to read medical books, even if only to see what doctors are reading. Go along to your local medical library — get a booklist from the nearest medical or university bookshop. The following shops will send a booklist if you send a stamped addressed envelope:

Family Planning Bookshop, 27-35 Mortimer Street, London W1A 4QW.

Compendium Bookshop, 24 Camden High Street, London NW1 (has books from the USA).

Rising Free, 182 Upper Street, London N1 (also has books from the USA).

National Childbirth Trust, 9 Queensborough Terrace, London W2 3TB.

We can send you a speculum for 50p including postage and we would like to hear from you with any comments or queries you may have. Write to us c/o Virago, 4th floor, 5 Wardour Street, London W1V 3HE.